# LOLA SINELLI

*Learn the secrets of permanent weight loss, reducing your dependency on sugar and starch, selling yourself, and getting anything you want!*

# Wants, Needs, and More...

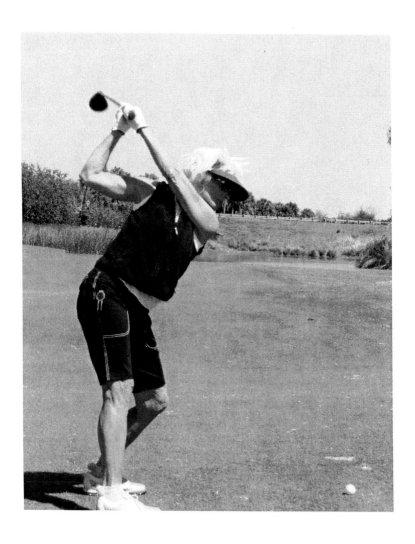

# about the author

Lola Sinelli is sixty-four years old and has been a fitness enthusiast and athlete for over forty years. She is also an artist. She ran competitively for ten years, did aerobics for ten years, played first base on coed softball teams, played tennis and racquetball for fifteen years, skied for twenty years, and golfed for fourteen years. She is the Fiddlers Creek Golf and Country Club's 2008, 2009, and 2010 Woman's Club champion. She is also Western Golf and Country Club's 2010 Woman's Club Champion. This book draws from her life experiences.

At the age of thirty-four, she began her best job—working as one of the first personal trainers in the club industry; she progressed to sales manager for the remainder of her fitness-related career. She helped build memberships in one of the top ten sport and fitness complexes in the country. She works out regularly by power walking, lifting weights, her own stretching/yoga program, and golfing several days a week. She is known affectionately by the name "Rocket" on the beach at Marco Island, Florida.

Her favorite song is "Whatever Lola Wants, Lola Gets."

www.wantsneedsandmore.com

In this book is a compilation of Lola's opinions and observations that are based on real life experiences and knowledge. She is not a medical doctor, and her suggestions should be used at your own risk.

ISBN: 1453652914
ISBN-13: 9781453652916
Library of Congress Control Number: 2010909392

# donation

∾

I am donating one dollar from each book to the Mathew Kind Recovery Fund.

Mat is a friend of mine who, at the young age of forty, had a very serious accident that thankfully spared his life but left him in a wheelchair. He is tremendously challenged each and every day. He just got married and is starting a new chapter in his life. Love to you Mat, always. My hope is that I sell millions of copies, to help with your ongoing physical therapy.

# dedication

This book is dedicated to my fantastic husband, Tom, for whom I patiently waited and wasn't sure I would ever meet; my mom, who taught me class, style, and generosity—she was my best friend, whom I dearly love and miss every day; to my dad, who taught me how to handle money and encouraged me to save and not spend—luckily I found someone very much like him; my daughters, Mrs. Nicole Lee (and David), Mrs. Jana Mattheu (and Jim); and my sons, Todd Matthews, Scott Sinelli (and Lillian), and Marc Sinelli, who are all my dear friends.

# acknowledgements

෨

A special thank you to Peggy Spano, who read a draft of this book and encouraged me to continue writing; to Tina, my sister-in-law, who was more interested in taking pictures while on our golf course than in golfing (the pictures on the course are hers); and my son-in-law David, who was kind enough to take the time to make me look as good as possible with his photographic skills.

Also, God bless our country and all our sons and daughters who fight to keep our wonderful nation safe and free.

Learn How to Lose Weight and Keep It Off for Good

Learn the Secrets of Getting What You Want

Learn the Secrets to Reducing Your
Dependency on Sugar and Starch

Learn How to Quit Smoking, Keep the
Weight off, and Never Start Smoking Again

Learn the Secrets of How to Sell Yourself

Learn the Meaning of True Fitness

Learn How to Go into Old Age with
Less Pain and More Flexibility

And Much, Much More

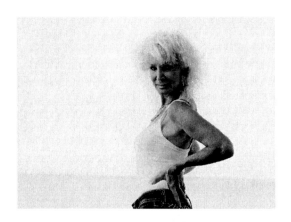

# table of contents

❧

# preface

I originally wanted to write a book about weight loss and how to be successful at it. During this process, I realized that to be successful at weight loss, you have to be successful, period. Successful people accomplish whatever they want. I wrote this book to give you the tools to help you become whatever and whomever you want. During the process of writing the book, I realized that I have much valuable health and wellness information that I could share with readers who would be interested in giving me a few hours of their time.

This is a self-help book to assist men and women in deciding what they want and need in life—and to get it! I have included many tips for a healthier, happier way of living.

I have chosen to include some pictures that I took of my favorite sunsets. In the beginning of each chapter, they are there to remind you at days end to reject all your bad habits and negative thinking, and begin each new day with great, new, positive awakenings.

The last picture is of the full moon, which, in astrology, governs the subconscious mind and is there to remind you that each new moon is a new beginning and a new ending.

**GOOD JUDGEMENT COMES FROM EXPERIENCE, AND EXPERIENCE COMES FROM BAD JUDGEMENT**

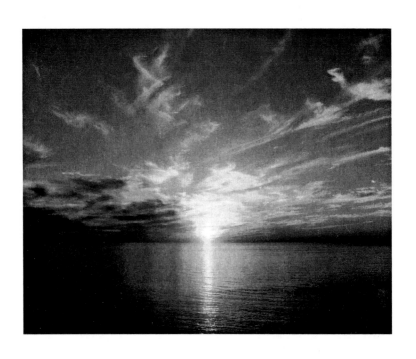

# chapter 1

# DEFINING YOUR WANTS AND NEEDS

*discipline is power*

❧

The hardest thing you will have to do during the reading of this book is to define and write down your **wants and needs**. I'll bet you can't do it right now. But, hopefully, by the end of this reading, you will know exactly what they are and how to get them.

When I first questioned my wants and needs, I was thirty-four years old and had never given it a thought. It took me five years to answer the question. I had all the necessities: food, clothing, a job, roof over my head, and two young children.

I'd left my husband of fourteen years, and I was a single parent and on my own for the first time in my life. I immediately got work as a waitress in a crummy restaurant and moved in with my parents...well, it was almost getting out on my own. My husband was verbally and physically abusive, so my self-esteem was so low that it was nonexistent. It was then that I began to learn how to go after what I wanted and deserved.

In July 1982, I was having my handwriting analyzed at some kind of holistic fair, and during the reading, one of the things the reader told me was to define my

**wants and needs**. I hated my waitressing job and luckily got fired, which opened the door to a whole new life. (I will share with you later the new life that opened up for me after being fired.) I learned from the experience of losing my job that you should never ever be afraid of change because it is the only way we grow. Still, I couldn't believe that *I* got fired! I was never very good at waitressing and learned later in life that I had strengths but waitressing wasn't one of them.

It took years to try to answer the question of what my **wants and needs** were, and I was so puzzled as to why I couldn't answer such an easy question. I thought about it all the time, but couldn't come up with an answer. What were my **wants and needs**? Was it a career? Was it fitness? Was it a man? No, it couldn't be a man. I just got rid of a man, so for sure it wasn't a man. Or was it?

*discipline is power*

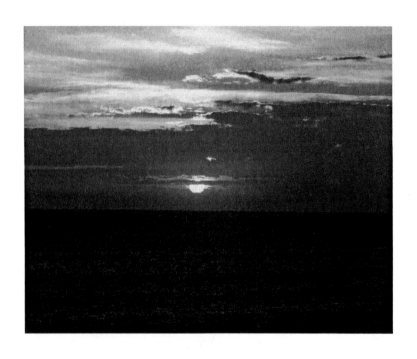

chapter 2:

# WANTS

*discipline is power*

∽

Fast-forward a few years, and after not wanting a man for any reason and still pondering the question of what my **wants and needs** were, I came to the decision that if I wanted a man, I should decide what kind of man I wanted. I knew I needed someone I could make a nice home with, and who could provide me with the tremendous security that I had as a child. Possibly for you, it would be a man or woman who could provide you with the security that you never had as a child.

I had decided that the men we all want must have these qualities:

1. Good to our family and children
2. Responsible
3. Dependable
4. Generous
5. Ambitious
6. Respectful to us
7. Kind
8. Loving
9. Good sense of humor
10. Likes dogs and cats

11. Good looking in our eyes
12. Must have a fitness lifestyle in my eyes
13. Hair—pretty dumb, I know, but I liked hair on a man's head. Looking back on this one, it was rather stupid because I now know many men who look great bald and balding.

My wants were not only about a man, but before you have a want, you have to assess your needs. A **want** is a desire or a lust for something. A **need** is something of necessity and an imperative requirement.

At the time, my need was a job and, luckily, I was at the right place at the right time and a job was put in my path. So my needs, at the moment, were taken care of.

However, most people don't even think about what they want. If you don't know what you want, you can't figure out how to get it. You must lay out a plan to get whatever your long-term wants are. That doesn't mean that it is all right to go out and put everything you want on a credit card. I am not talking about immediate gratification or impulse spending. My very smart dad taught me if you can't afford it, **don't buy it,** save for it. You will appreciate it more. Unfortunately, in this day and age, credit cards are way too easy to accumulate. Just start college and see how many applications you get! My generation never had credit cards growing up, so we had to **save** for everything we wanted or needed.

I want you to start thinking about what you really want in this lifetime. Where do you want to be at thirty, forty, fifty, etc.? What kind of a person do you want to spend these years with? What work do you want to do, so you can prepare yourself for the life you want? What are your strengths? Start thinking about that right now. So many people just flail through life without ever preparing for it, but it is so important to figure out early what your strengths are, so that you can be good at your work and love what you do for the money you make. You will be a much happier person.

*discipline is power*

chapter 3:

# AFFIRMATIONS

*discipline is power*

ᖪᖣ

After three or four years, I still had not found the answer to what my **wants and needs** were. But I think I was getting closer.

The first time I ever heard the word **AFFIRMATION** was from my friend Colleen, who sold Amway products with her husband in the '80s. Through their training, they were taught how affirmations work. You set goals and reach them through writing them down and putting them in a place where you see them several times a day. By repeating them out loud over and over and over, you accentuate the positive changes for which you are wishing. An example would be something like this: "I am a great salesperson. I am smart, I am funny, and I am well-liked."

The whole idea behind affirmations is what the mouth speaks, the mind hears. You can be assured that, after a while, you will be a great salesperson who is smart, funny, and well-liked. You reinforce these words over and over and, in time, you will become what you think you are. You become what your mind hears you speak.

I want you to memorize these phrases: **WHAT THE MOUTH SPEAKS, THE MIND HEARS.** This is extremely important, so listen to the words that come out

9

of your mouth because **WHETHER YOU THINK YOU CAN OR YOU THINK YOU CAN'T, YOU'RE RIGHT!** In other words, what you think you can accomplish, you will accomplish. If you dwell in self pity you will never know joy. The mind is a powerful tool, and positive thinking can help you get whatever you **want and need**.

I want you to take a minute to think about some of the things that come out of your mouth regularly. When you speak to your friends or relatives, what kind of things do you say? Are some of them negative? Is your mouth repeatedly speaking things like "I can't get the job," "I can't stop overeating," "I am a loser," or "I can't find a man"? What do you think is going to happen if this goes on day after day? You will *never* get the job, stop overeating, or find a man. **YOU WILL FAIL AT EVERYTHING.**

You are programming yourself for failure every time you open your mouth and berate yourself or your life. The first thing you must start doing right now is never, ever say the word *can't*. Don't even think that you can't and never say that you can't.

The first man I dated after my divorce was a very nice Romeo kind of guy; he was the one who taught me never to say *can't*, and I will never forget him because of this very important lesson. (Thanks Bob.) Remember, **if you think you can or if you think you can't, you are right**. Replace *can't* with *can*: "I *can* do it," "I *will* do it," and "I *am* capable of doing it." **NEVER, EVER SAY *CAN'T*.**

Writing down affirmations and saying them over and over got me my wants and needs, and it will do the same for you. You need to be what you want to be, and you have to define it and want it badly enough to work at getting it. Be prepared to receive what you want. Do your homework to help get you there.

What will your affirmations be? Write them down right now.

_____

_____

_____

_____

_____

_____

Now rip these out and tape them to your mirror, so they remind you every day to say them out loud, over and over.

*discipline is power*

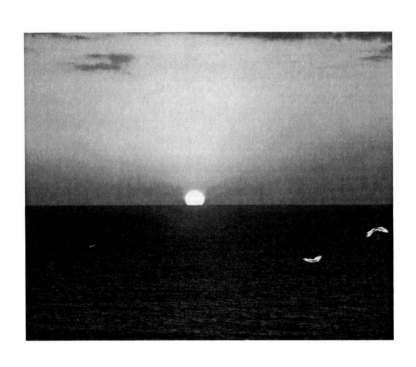

# chapter 4:

# TOOLS

*discipline is power*

༄

The Oxford English Dictionary defines a tool as "a hand instrument, a mechanical device, a servile helper." To get what you want, you have to have the tools.

Anyone can get whatever they want. If an individual is well dressed and looks impressive, he will get what he wants if he believes he can. **"If he believes he can"** are the key words. Since I learned to apply this to my own life, I have gotten everything I have ever wanted. The hard part is deciding what I wanted.

One important tool we have is our looks. Society works on appearances and first impressions.  If you are single, try to be as attractive as possible each day because you never know whom you will meet. If you are married, keep your spouse interested by taking care of your appearance. You lazy people know who you are! Men, please trim your nose hairs and get your eyebrows trimmed. I have seen some men who look like cartoon characters. Come on, you guys—look in the mirror! Women are lucky; we have makeup to help us look good, but you men don't get any help at all. **SUCCESS IS WHEN PREPARATION AND OPPORTUNITY MEET.** Taking care of your appearance is a small price to pay for success. You may not be in total control of everything, but you are in total control of your appearance.

The first tool you need is the best hairdresser you can find. Both men and women need great stylists. Not all hairdressers are excellent at color and styling. Do your homework. When you see someone with a great color or style, stop them and ask who did their hair then write it down immediately. The person will be flattered, and you will find someone good at the same time. Men, forget about coloring your hair. I have never met a man who looks good with colored hair. You guys just look better slowly graying.

If you are a woman and your face is square, you need a style that balances out the square jaw. If your face is round, you probably need bangs to break up the roundness. If your face is oval, a short, cropped style would be good. Second, get a color that complements your skin tones and doesn't detract from your face. When your hair color is right, you'll know it; your eyes will sparkle and your skin will look good. When it's wrong, your complexion will look sallow or sickly. Believe me, you don't want to walk around looking sickly and have people asking you if you are feeling well.

Usually, at better salons, they have makeup artists. Spend a few bucks to see what kind of look they can give you. Remember, they are professionals. It may take you a few days to get used to the changes because instinctively no one likes change, but change is always good. **You only grow when you change**. Growth is always good when you are trying to get what you want. Hair salons have very creative artists, and for a small price, they can make you bloom. Women get stuck in time warps. You've seen them: the ratted hair and blue eye shadows from the '60s. Oops, the blue eye shadow is back but it's important to keep your hair style fashionable.

When I started graying, stylists talked me into doing a base color and highlights. The base looked good for two days and then washed me out, and instinctively I knew it was wrong, but I didn't know why. So for three weeks, I would walk around feeling like my colors weren't right. When my daughter finally became a stylist, she suggested thirty-volume peroxide and no base color, with lots of highlights. Voilá—that was the right thing for my skin tone. Now I do my own color and cut, and save lots of money. I started cutting my dolls' hair when I was little and always loved doing makeovers for my friends; we had such fun getting beautiful!

Update your look regularly by looking at fashion magazines. That doesn't mean that you have to do whatever they say, but maybe just create your own style, which is updated and comfortable for you. Most times I look in those magazines, I think to myself, "*Who walks around looking like that?*" I think it is more fantasy than anything, but you can get some good ideas for putting together the clothes in your own closet. Personally, I like shoes and purses; you can update any outfit with new shoes and a cute purse.

Get to know what colors look best on you. Go to **colormebeautiful.com.** The book *Color Me Beautiful* came out in the '80s and gives you all the tools that will help you decide which colors work for you. You are classified as a spring, summer, winter, or autumn. The book tells you your wearable colors depending on your eye color, hair color, and skin color. It is a foolproof way of picking clothing that will match everything in your closet—and even your hair color. I am a winter and can wear pure white, true grays, black, navy, royal blue, light yellow, turquoise, emerald green, and pink. Copyright laws prevent me from going into great detail; however, if you go to the Web site, you will find out what your season is. Maybe from this basic description you can tell if you are a winter by knowing that these colors look good on you. Try putting some of the other colors in your season up to your face, and you may be surprised how good they make you look. Try putting the wrong season up to your face, and you can see how horrible they make you look.

My mom, who had excellent taste, would always buy me the cutest tops. Occasionally she would show up with a blouse that was stunning. I would put it on, and even as cute as it was, it just never looked right on me. This went on for years, and those tops stayed unworn in my closet year after year. Eventually I would give them to my friend Barbara, who was a redhead (and whom I later found out was an autumn). They would look stunning on her, and she loved my mom's taste. When *Color Me Beautiful* came out, I finally realized I was a winter, and everything my mom bought me was for an autumn. A redhead looks great in the olives and beiges which were the colors my mom bought me. Those colors washed me out. Instinctively I knew they looked wrong, but I never knew why. Now, in my later years, I am an artist, love decorating, and have flair with color. Back then, I knew the colors were wrong but didn't know why. My mom was also wearing all the wrong colors. We both finally learned what our colors were, and then she quit buying me stuff. I am not sure why. I should have asked her that one!

In her later years in the retirement home, people always commented on how wonderful my mother looked. She always had on the right colors and wore a perfect lipstick color. She looked wonderful every day—every single day! It was harder for her as she aged, but each day she tried, and it made her feel good when people noticed.

Almost everyone has heard of *Extreme Makeover*; it was hit show for a few seasons. My suggestion is if there is something on your face that is borderline scary, beg, or borrow the money to get it fixed. After all, the first thing people see is your face and your smile. Make it so you will be pleasing to look at because it will be the best investment in your future that you will ever make. Most plastic surgeons have payment plans of some sort or can set you up with a bank at a good interest rate, so take advantage of it. Make sure they are board certified in plastic surgery and see the before-and-after pictures of their patients.

I finally had my nose fixed at the age of thirty-eight. I grew up not being able to breathe because of a deviated septum, and I was teased unmercifully by one of my brothers because of the shape of my nose. My lips were always dry and cracked, and I was miserable. I begged my mom to get it fixed my whole life, and all she would say is that it was a classic Roman nose. It was classic all right—it was a classic nose that was hooked and bumpy!

I would say, "But, Mom, I can't breathe." She never heard that part. My name was not Lola growing up; it was Eagle Beak and Pelican Face. Thanks to my little brother who came up with those names—can you guess that we never got along as children? I had a few names for him, too. He had an automatic nose job when we were playing monkey in the middle, and the hardball thrown by my neighbor who was seven years older than us, ticked my shoulder and bounced in his face, splattering his nose all over it. I think the plastic surgeon was a much easier way to go. Now, thinking back, I realize how those names had a very strong impact on how much I really hated my nose. Now, years later, my little brother and I are terrific friends.

When I turned thirty-eight, one of the young girls with whom I worked (who was not very attractive and a little frumpy) went on vacation for two weeks and had her nose fixed, got a chin implant, had her braces removed, and got a new hair color and style. When I first saw her, I was stunned. She looked beautiful. Better yet, she was beaming. You could see it in her personality and newfound confidence. She smiled all the time. She knew how good she looked, and I knew how good she felt. She put the frumpy years behind her, and it opened up a whole new life for her. That day, I made an appointment with the same surgeon. In August1987, I underwent the surgery I had wanted my whole life. It was not pleasant by any means, but it changed my life.

People had always used the term *attractive* when referring to my looks. I never, ever believed it because what I saw in the mirror was my brother sitting on my shoulder, calling me Eagle Beak and Pelican Face; I never saw an attractive person. I only saw a great big nose. All of a sudden, people started telling me I was so pretty. Who, me? Me? You talking to me? Yeah! Somebody thought I was pretty! I met my husband six months later. He was my **want,** and I was prepared to meet him. He is perfect for me. He fills every want I had on my list. He is a drop-dead handsome Marlboro Man-type. I didn't even realize that the famous "man list" had been fulfilled until many years later, when I came across it. I thought to myself, *Subconsciously, I got what I wanted; I just had to write it down and ask for it.*

As for the rest of one's appearance, what can be done for your smile today is amazing. When you smile, people notice your teeth. Make sure they are beautiful. Find a cosmetic dentist in your area and get prices for repair work, then get a second opinion, and work one against the other. They will cut their prices if asked. They can change the shape, the bite, the color, and the width of your smile. Try to make your face look like it could launch a thousand ships or at least a few hundred. Make sure the changes are up to your standards before they cement them in because they are permanent.

Teeth whiteners are everywhere, in every drug store you frequent, and they work. So spend the money on your teeth because it is important. You can see that when people have white teeth, they are more confident.

If you are an adult with acne, get it treated. If you are a teenager suffering with bad skin, beg, beg, beg your parents to take you to the dermatologist for treatment. Bad skin can be helped. Try going to a reputable facialist because something, somewhere, can be done. Maybe just Retinol a few nights a week will do the trick. Nobody likes to look at disgusting pimples, and the damage they do to teenagers is, in some cases, never repaired. All of us can improve our looks, no matter what God gave us. Remember, God also gave us the tools to improve ourselves!

Your face is your most important tool. Skin care is critical. **Stay out of the sun** and **DON'T SMOKE**. This is the best advice I can give you. A tan is not attractive when the underlying damage is either skin cancer or early wrinkles. The sun's UV radiation causes collagen to break down at a higher rate than just with normal aging. Skin cancer could mean they have to cut a big chunk of your face off, so you don't die. Tanning booths come with warnings; heed those cancer warnings. Just recently I read the following study:

> The findings back up previous indications that sunbathing, both artificial and the real thing, can be habit-forming. A small 2006 study found that those who persistently visit tanning beds can experience withdrawal symptoms if they don't get their UV-high. And a 2008 study revealed that about 18 percent of outdoor tanners qualified as addicted. (Ultraviolet, or UV, rays emitted by the sun are what cause sunburns). The results of the current work, which is based on a larger sample and possibly more robust research methods, also suggest that reducing the risky behavior might take more than just public awareness campaigns. For some, it might require interventions more along the lines of what's used as treatment for substance abusers.  Can you believe it?

The study is published in the April issue of *Archives of Dermatology*, a journal of the American Medical Association. That's all we need: something else to get addicted to. Ugh!

My husband had to get a big chunk taken out of his nose because of skin cancer. They replaced it with a skin graft taken from his shoulder. He had thirteen stitches in his shoulder, and it was a pretty depressing surgery. At one of our appointments with his surgeon, a man came in the waiting area with no nose at all. He had only a bandage over what used to be his nose. I was pretty horrified, and my heart went out to that poor man. Not an appealing thing to think about. If you are lucky, your face will last eighty-plus years or so, and you want to look as good as you can whether you are eighteen or eighty.

There are many fake tan products and bronzers out there that can give you the appearance of a tan; try them if you want to be tan or try a tinted moisturizer with sunscreen. Have you ever noticed the people who live in L.A. who aren't actresses or models or who live in Florida? Women in their late twenties look like they are ten years older. They are exposed to the sun daily and cannot escape it. Walk the beach in Florida and see some of the alligator skin I see daily. I always try to walk very early. Try to cover your skin because sunscreen can only help prevent skin cancer not premature aging.

There are experts who question whether sunscreen helps prevent cancer. We do need sun for our vitamin D levels, so safe sun, not overexposure, is good for us. Vitamin D is known as the sunshine vitamin because it is created in the body when we are exposed to sunlight.

The experts say morning sun and late afternoon sun are the safest times to be exposed, always avoiding 11:00 a.m. to 3:00 p.m. Cover your skin with scarves, long sleeves, and hats; if you golf, wear gloves on both hands. The skin care you get at the dermatologist office or the plastic surgeons office-the lasers, the dermabrasions, and other things are there if you have the money. If by chance you have abused your face and are now ready to start repair work, but don't want that costly and invasive face lift, there is another way. For a number of years, Dr. J. William Little of Washington D.C. has stressed the importance of filling out the hollows of the face and adding volume where it has been lost. He calls this volumetric rejuvenation. Many plastic surgeons today achieve volumetric rejuvenation by injecting your own fat into the face rather than using synthetic fillers which are usually only temporary.

Dr. Stanley P. Gulin of Naples, FL carries it one step further. He combines the fat with platelet rich plasma obtained from a small amount of blood. The fat actually contains stem cells and the platelet plasma has growth factors so the combination not only gives the necessary volume to the face but also revitalizes the skin. He calls this a stem cell liquid facelift. It can be done either alone or in combination with a facelift avoiding that pulled or stretched look. This is why many of the older movie stars look so good at sixty five and seventy five.

*discipline is power*

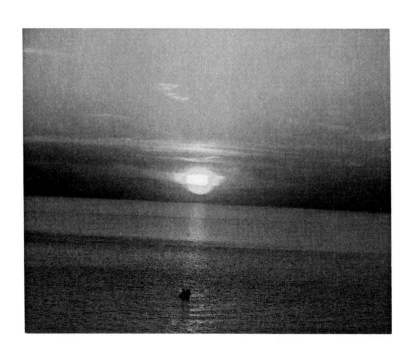

# chapter 5:

# SELLING YOURSELF

*discipline is power*

༄

In sales, the first thing you have to do is sell yourself. People will like you more if you ask them questions about themselves. Everyone loves talking about himself. Do you realize that people have three to seven nos? They will say no three to seven times before they say yes. If you are in sales, you need to know this. Remember when you were trying to talk your parents into something, and they would say no over and over? If you were persistent enough you could get them to say yes. My kids always did this to me and because of this, they are very strong adults.

Secondly, if you have unpleasant looks, you won't be able to sell anything as well as if your looks are pleasing. All of us in one way or another are in sales. We sell ourselves as friends, lovers, and businesspeople. Maybe we are not all commissioned salespeople, but we are selling ourselves every day. Just think for a moment about a good-looking man you know with perfect white teeth and trimmed eyebrows and nose hairs. Picture his face and smile. Now picture him with yellow teeth, hair coming out of his nose, and wiry, inch-long eyebrows. How appealing does he look? What a difference!

The same can be done with weight. Just picture someone you know with a weight problem and how they would look at their normal weight; think about how they would feel about themselves and how differently they would relate to people if they were at an ideal weight.

The hit TV program *The Biggest Loser* is a perfect example. You see the participants in the beginning, very obese and very sad; they are all so helpless, scared, and pitiful. They are all there begging for change, even though they know it will be extremely difficult. You then see them going through the process of changing their lifestyle, being browbeaten into changing their habits, and losing weight in exchange for a large sum of money if they win. They are eliminated one by one, week after week if they are the slowest loser, and, finally, the last show of the season, there is a winner. At the end of the show, the winner emerges a normal size and is beaming with pride and feeling terrific about the end result of all the hard work. They winner is presented with a large check; your large check could and would be a brand new, happier, and more fulfilled life.

I stopped at the drugstore yesterday to get some pictures developed. The woman behind the counter was at least three hundred and fifty pounds and about five-foot-two. She was in a store uniform that was two sizes too small. She could hardly look at me when I started talking to her. She may have been embarrassed because of my size. She was very nice, and all I could think was *"Is she in pain? Is that how she got so heavy? Was she under tremendous stress? What would be the reason she would let herself get out of control? How did she get that big?"* I was very sweet to her, and we exchanged some small talk. By making her smile, I know that I brightened her day. She could look me in the eyes and was happier when I left. *I made a difference.* We have to have compassion for the morbidly obese; look *at* them instead of looking away. Some of them don't want to be noticed for some reason or another. Many have been abused, many have no education on health or nutrition, and others have had a horrible family life. If you see them on the street, and your eyes meet, smile at them. They could really use a smile.

The point is that a big part of selling yourself and having confidence has to do with appearances. Have you ever gone to buy a car, walked into a dealership, and everyone was too busy to talk to you? You had a chance to walk around looking at the cars in the showroom and also to look at all the salespeople. You knew who you wanted to help you before anyone came over. You wanted the better-looking ones or the one that looked the best. You wanted the man with the handsome suit on or the woman with the nice hair and beautiful scarf. That man and that woman are the people you want to have a business relationship with. This is why you have to look as polished and as professional as you can, specifically for this reason. You want more people to be attracted to you rather than to someone else, so *you* can get what *you* **want** and **need**.

Personally, whenever I buy a car, I always seek out a woman. I guess it's because, in business, I always had a hard time because I was a woman in a man's world. I will never forget being at my job and asking a higher-up which one of my male superiors was the male chauvinist pig: Was it the owner or the general manager? He looked me straight in the eyes and said "Lola, it's the world." In the late '80s, he was so right.

We took our car into the dealership for service the other day, and I wandered into the new car area to peek. Right away this cute little darling of a girl came up to me and introduced herself, and we had a very nice conversation. Guess where I am going to buy my next car and from whom?

*discipline is power*

chapter 6:

# THE BODY: ANOTHER
# IMPORTANT TOOL

*discipline is power*

∾

Now, understand...I am a nobody. I am a loving wife and mother, and a giving daughter and friend. The people who know me, besides my inner circle of friends and family, are the thousands of people who have found a healthier lifestyle because of my work. I am not a celebrity who has a personal trainer or gets one three months before a movie or a personal appearance. I am just like you—a regular person who learned to take advantage of the tools that were out there to better my life. Ultimately you are responsible for the way you project yourself to humanity, however good or bad it may be.

In the mid-'80s to mid-'90s, I worked for one of the top ten health and sport complexes in the country. I was the sales manager for the last nine years and a personal fitness trainer for the first two years. In an average month, I signed up thirty to seventy-five people, and helped change their lives. They were begging and pleading for a healthier way of life and slimmer bodies. The most successful of them were the hardest people to sell. Sometimes it took years and seven nos to get a prospective member to make the commitment to fitness, but they were the most appreciative and put in the most effort.

We had twenty indoor tennis courts, twenty racquetball courts, squash, aerobics, spinning, three thousand square feet of fitness, indoor and outdoor pools, kids' area, a bar, and a restaurant. It was before its time, and I helped build the membership to over six thousand. I stayed there so long that I signed up the same people over and over. It was a facility that was two hundred and fifty thousand square feet—all of it indoors. It was there, in 1985, that I started to educate myself about the human body.

I heard every excuse in the world about why people couldn't join, but the truth was that they were all *afraid of failure*. They were the ones who would say to themselves and to me, "I can't do this," "I don't have the time," "I don't have the money," or "I have to check with my husband." Others were too passive to take any action to change their lives. Remember: **WHAT THE MOUTH SPEAKS, THE MIND HEARS**. If you say these things out loud, and you believe them, there will be no change. I just hope that some of these people joined other clubs or turned to fitness and health before heart trouble, high blood pressure, cancer, stroke, diabetes, bad knees/ankles/hips/feet, or death. Sometimes, being a salesperson, I could spark the right conversations or paint the right picture of fitness for people, and they would jump at the chance to change their lives. I always felt sorry for the ones I lost. Good intentions won't get you anything. **Action gets you what you want**. Remember, we are fighting disease every day of our lives.

If you can squeeze in twenty minutes of exercise three times a week, you can initiate weight loss. A calorie is a pre-SI metric unit of energy. There are thirty-five hundred calories in a pound. You need the heat of exercise to burn off the calories. If you ate the same number of calories and only exercised twenty minutes, three times per week, you would lose approximately one pound in seven weeks just from exercising. The seven weeks will go by whether you exercise or not. I know seven weeks is a long time to lose a pound, but it's better than gaining. It will give you the initiative to exercise more and more—and the more you exercise, the more you will go for healthier, low-calorie foods.

After a while, you will look at the calories in a serving of something and calculate the number of calories needed to burn it off. "*Hmm, that will take forty-five minutes on the bike to work off, at four hundred and fifty calories an hour, or one hour of fast walking for five hundred calories.*" You will start to think twice about putting that item in your mouth. Maybe then you will just take a bite and throw the rest away. This, by the way, is a very good method. I use it all the time.

*discipline is power*

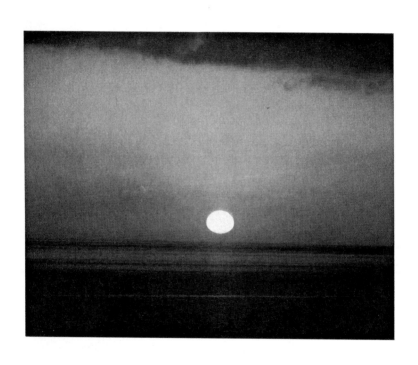

# chapter 7

# HEALTH

*discipline is power*

෨

Can we talk about the healthier foods part of the last chapter for a minute? Think about this: Our immune system is our most powerful protector, so if we feed ourselves well, we are feeding our immune system to help fight disease. Health begins at the cellular level and continues through the body. If you feed yourself, you will live. If you feed your cells, you will live better and longer. Do you want to just feed yourself or do you want to really *feed* yourself? Again, we are all fighting disease every single day of our lives. For example, nitrates, which are preservatives that are used in meats, bacon, hot dogs, and many other foods, can be converted by the body to a powerful cancer-causing chemical according to the Web site *time to run.com*. I have tried to keep my family away from all forms of luncheon meats and cured meats, always trying to eat only natural peanut butter in sandwiches. Some processed meats still use nitrates for preservatives, and it's been thirty-five years. Be careful what you put into your mouth and the mouths of your family. The trap that we all fall into is eating for reasons other than health: social eating, comfort eating, boredom eating, misery eating, and stress eating.

Remember, healthy people have an edge in business, home life, and in everything they do because they *feel* better.

In my thirty-five-plus years of experience in health and weight reduction, I have read countless books on how to lose weight and on optimum health and nutrition. Some seem to have some kind of a gimmick. I have been involved with every form of exercise since the mid-'60s. Being the sales manager at the fitness complex where I worked helped me get and stay in shape. It changed my life and brought me closer to my **wants** and **needs**. This is where my future sent me after I got fired from the crummy restaurant.

The first book I ever read about health was *Sugar Blues* by William Dufty, which was published in 1975. I loved that book and learned so much from it; after that, I couldn't read enough books about our bodies. Dufty said sugar was poison, and America didn't really have heart disease until we started importing sugar. Of course, our life expectancy back in the 1800s or early 1900s was about fifty or fifty-five; our technology today is so wonderful, thankfully, which is why we all live longer. If you have a pain in your chest, you dial 911 and shortly thereafter the paramedics arrive, give you fluids and medication, and transport you to the hospital to avert a heart attack. There they do a few tests and tell you that you need a heart catherization to clear your arteries of blockages, need a stent to keep your artery open, or need open-heart bypass surgery. This is the result of advances in medical knowledge and technology. Isn't technology wonderful? There were no paramedics, ambulances, or state-of-the-art technology in the 1800s or early 1900s, and you would be dead. I have a few friends who were lucky enough to listen to their bodies and at young ages averted death, one with stents, and one with bypass surgery, and they are both alive and well today.

I agree with Dufty. Sugar *is* poison. According to Ann Louise Gittleman, author of *How to Stay Young and Healthy in a Toxic World*, "Sugar is **not** an innocent substance that gives us pleasure and causes no harm. Quite the contrary; there is perhaps nothing else in the diet that promotes disease and aging more over the long term than excess sugar." Withdrawal-like symptoms can occur when sugar is eliminated from your diet, as I experienced on more than one occasion. (I will expound on this later.)

After reading *Sugar Blues*, I realized that I had a new passion. I started gleaning from books everything I could about health and nutrition, and decided that these were going to be the years I concentrated on bettering myself.

*discipline is power*

# chapter 8

# WEIGHT LOSS

*discipline is power*

❧

Weight loss is just a matter of mathematics, which, by the way, was my worst subject. It is so simple—and if I can figure it out, so can you.

If your goal weight is one hundred and thirty pounds, you add one zero to the one hundred and thirty for a total of thirteen hundred calories. These are the amount of calories that you can consume daily to get to your goal. If you exercise thirty minutes a day, you burn off, depending on your size and intensity of your workout, approximately two hundred and fifty calories. Add that to the thirteen hundred calories, and your total caloric intake should be no more than fifteen hundred and fifty calories per day. This is for daily maintenance. My word, is that easy or what? If you exercise less or eat more you will gain weight. If you exercise more and eat less, you will lose weight.

A pound is thirty-five hundred calories. If you have five pounds to lose, you have to cut calories by seventeen thousand and five hundred—that is five pounds times thirty-five hundred calories in a pound, which equals seventeen thousand and five hundred. In thirty days, if you cut your calories by five hundred and eighty-three per day, you would lose five pounds. If you want to burn off those five hundred and eighty-three calories, get moving, walk an hour or walk a half an hour and cut the calories by half.

I have known this for thirty years and it has been confirmed by Professor Mark Haub, a professor of human nutrition at Kansas State University. He began eating twinkies, nutty bars, powdered donuts, and Doritos to prove that weight loss is just about calorie counting. He kept his calories to 1,800 per day and lost twenty-seven pounds in two months. His bad cholesterol dropped by twenty percent and his good cholesterol increased by twenty percent. Calorie counting works.

Get a little booklet or go on the Web and read the caloric value of different foods, and get a small scale to weigh your food so you have an exact count. Also, use the Web to find out what exercise burns off how many calories per hour for your weight and size. Try to eliminate or at least cut back the white stuff— breads, flour, sugar, potatoes, rice, and pasta. Once you eat them your body will turn them to sugar and want more. And, for goodness sake, get off of regular sugar. If you are addicted to sugar, which I have been two times in my life, I will tell you how to be free of your addiction later. When I finally gave up most, not all, of the white stuff, I found true weight maintenance. It is a wonderful feeling not to have to diet or battle that scale every day. Exert the energy and then you can relax more about what you put into your mouth.

Remember, those thirty days will pass whether you are counting calories or not. If you want to lose weight more quickly, cut your calories, and increase your activity. The "experts" say we shouldn't drop our daily caloric intake lower than twelve hundred for women and fifteen hundred for men since you could put your body into starvation mode, and your metabolism would be compromised. I don't agree and have always eaten less than twelve hundred calories to lose quicker however, they are the "experts."

You must keep a log and a running total as you eat each day. It's the best way to keep track of everything you eat. Also, drink water. Keep a glass of water close by and drink eight to ten glasses every day; it will fill you up and help flush out the fat. Don't drink more than eight to ten glasses because it could be dangerous to your health. Try not to use bottled water because it contains BPA, a very controversial chemical and may even be banned by the Canadian government according to an article in the *New York Times* dated April 16, 2008. I have heard that it takes two years to get bottled water to the consumer; whether it's true or not, I don't know, but, if so, where have all those plastic bottles been stored for two years: in a hot warehouse or a frozen one? Their ingredients could be even more dangerous. Think about what you put in your mouth each day and track it.

Don't let yourself get so hungry that you stop on the way home and gorge. Eat smaller meals more frequently to keep your metabolism raised and burning more calories. Keep low-calorie snacks with you all the time. Every time you exercise, you will burn more calories throughout the day because exercise keeps your metabolism raised about 15 percent for the next ten to fifteen hours. Also, don't think *dieting*; think *healthy eating.* We all know what healthy eating is: veggies, salads, lean protein, and small amounts of starch or white stuff. Remember that starches turn into sugar, which will keep you craving sugar throughout the day. I recently have cut back on wheat, which, according to my nutritionist, is inflammatory to the system, and, I swear, whether it's in my mind or not, I feel better and have fewer aches and pains.

So, in review:

1. **KEEP A LOG AND ADD UP YOUR CALORIES AS YOU GO EACH DAY.**
2. **IN THE MORNING OR THE NIGHT BEFORE, PREPARE FOR WHAT YOU WILL EAT AT EACH MEAL.**
3. **EAT SMALLER, MORE FREQUENT MEALS TO KEEP YOUR METABOLISM UP.**
4. **DRINK EIGHT TO TEN GLASSES OF WATER DAILY TO KEEP YOUR BELLY FULL AND FLUSH FAT. MORE WATER MIGHT DAMAGE YOUR HEALTH, SO LIMIT YOURSELF TO TEN GLASSES.**
5. **STAY AWAY FROM STARCHES AND SUGARS. IF YOU MUST INDULGE, WAIT UNTIL EVENING AND HAVE ONLY A SMALL AMOUNT.**
6. **EXERCISE OFTEN AND FREQUENTLY, AND KEEP TRACK OF HOW MUCH YOU BURN OFF.**
7. **KEEP YOUR EATING TOTALS AT THE END OF THE DAY AND DEDUCT THE CALORIES YOU BURNED FROM EXERCISE.**

**Come on, it's just a little work, but the returns are very, very big.**

**Monday**                                          calories
    **Breakfast** _____    _____
    **Lunch** _____    _____
    **Snack** _____    _____
    **Dinner** _____    _____
    **Snack** _____    _____

**Tuesday**                                         calories
    **Breakfast** _____    _____
    **Lunch** _____    _____
    **Snack** _____    _____
    **Dinner** _____    _____
    **Snack** _____    _____

**Wednesday**                                       calories
    **Breakfast** _____    _____
    **Lunch** _____    _____
    **Snack** _____    _____
    **Dinner** _____    _____
    **Snack** _____    _____

**Thursday**                                        calories
    **Breakfast** _____    _____
    **Lunch** _____    _____
    **Snack** _____    _____
    **Dinner** _____    _____
    **Snack** _____    _____

**Friday**                                    **calories**
   **Breakfast** _____     _____
   **Lunch**     _____     _____
   **Snack**     _____     _____
   **Dinner**    _____     _____
   **Snack**     _____     _____

**Saturday**                                  **calories**
   **Breakfast** _____     _____
   **Lunch**     _____     _____
   **Snack**     _____     _____
   **Dinner**    _____     _____
   **Snack**     _____     _____

**Sunday**                                    **calories**
   **Breakfast** _____     _____
   **Lunch**     _____     _____
   **Snack**     _____     _____
   **Dinner**    _____     _____
   **Snack**     _____     _____

*discipline is power*

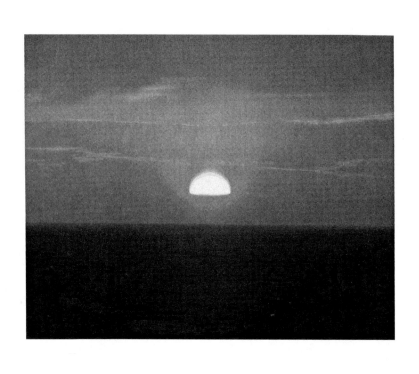

# chapter 9

# HEALTH CLUBS

*discipline is power*

∽

I learned so much from the people I talked to each day while selling memberships at my health club. I spent an average of twenty minutes to an hour or more with each prospect and made so many friends. Some of my oldest and dearest friends came from that job, like my wonderful husband, Tom, and my friend Colleen, as well as my interest in health and nutrition. Maybe that is why I worked there…to eventually write this book? Luckily, my husband came after a few exterior and interior improvements.

Joining a fitness club or a gym may be somewhat intimidating at first but stick with it. You will meet people and be more comfortable each time you go. Work with a personal trainer and he or she will introduce you to the members. Think of it as a growing experience to get to where you want to be, and smile at everyone. Smiling will be helpful to make new acquaintances. When I first started my job, I met Colleen, and she said she was interested in finding a workout partner, as was I. We still walk together quite often, and it is hard to believe that we met twenty-five years ago.

If you are very obese and afraid to go to a club, know that the people there will embrace you and encourage you, so do not be afraid. Also, get an okay from the doctor before starting any exercise regime.

*discipline is power*

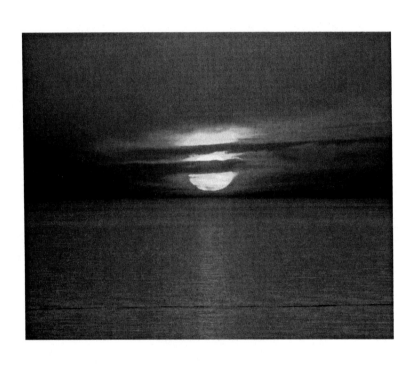

# chapter 10

# WORKING OUT

*discipline is power*

∞

I have been working out since I was twenty-one years old, and I have changed my thoughts as I have gone from my twenties to my sixties. I used to work out hard, lifting all that I could lift and running as fast as I could run. Neither of these activities ever made me lose weight. I only started losing weight when I started with the modified Adkins program or restricted my calories. Now that I am in my sixties, I realize that lighter weights and more repetitions are better than heavier weights, and power walking is better than running. I have had many injuries over the years, and I can pinpoint the exercises that injured me. I would like to pass along some of the exercises that cause injury to help you avoid the same problems.

Each injury took a minimum of one year to heal. The old saying that "the body can heal itself" is true, in most cases—only the older you get, the longer it takes. My elbow injury took the longest to heal, about five years. It was caused by bicep curls with too much weight. It was so painful that I couldn't grab a plate. I had six or seven cortisone shots, and they worked but were very painful. After I received a shot, the pain was gone, but it always came back within a few weeks or months, after I started working out again. I had to take a few years off of lifting for it to heal.

Also, don't get thrown out of a golf cart! That wasn't the first time my husband threw me out of a cart, but it took me a year and a half to recover after flipping end over end and rolling to a stop. He went one way, and I went the other way. I thought I was going to be paralyzed immediately after the fall and was very, very sore for a long time. Also, don't get hit with a golf cart, as I did. It took me four months to get over that one. Sit against the back cushion in golf carts, hold on to the handles, and, if you are a passenger, prop your foot up against the cart for stability. All golf carts come with warnings; they can be extremely dangerous.

**Power Walk**

Power walk rather than run. If you must run, switch off every other day with power walking. On my daily walks, I utilize my brain; no music—just thinking and spiritual time for me. You can't believe how many issues I conclude in my mind or how much anger I can rid myself of. Sometimes I am talking to myself and get caught by someone—very embarrassing. But it is vitally important to give back to ourselves because we are so busy making money, taking care of children, and doing for others that we forget that we need our time, too.

**Tricep Extension**

Do not do triceps extension exercises on a stationary station, with a great amount of weight, where you extend your arms straight out while your upper arms are supported by the machine. These types of tricep exercises stress the elbows and the ligaments going through them. You will probably get tennis elbow from them if you use heavy weights. Stop doing them immediately if your elbows start to hurt. This was the most common injury when I was a trainer. There are many other ways to do tricep exercises. Ask your trainer or look it up on the Web.

**Bicep Curls**

If you are doing single bicep curls, try to do them so that your body is supporting the sides of your arms as you lift the weights. This will take some of the pressure off your elbows. Also, when you begin doing this exercise, start with three-pound weights, for women, and let your elbows get used to the strain then move up to five pounds and then eight or ten after a few weeks. Men can start with eight- to ten-pound weights. I was surprised that after eliminating this exercise for years because of my elbow pain, when I began therapy for my golf cart injury, they started me out with two- or three-pound weights, and my elbows were fine. I now do twelve -pound bicep curls.

**Lateral Shoulder Raises**

If you are doing shoulder raises, do them with lighter weights. I injured my shoulder doing this exercise, and the only way to heal is to stop doing them and stretch your shoulder every which way. It is still annoying two years later, but therapeutic massage helped tremendously.

**Leg Extension**

This exercise can do injury to your knees, so I have eliminated it from my routine.

**Running**

Running is a great heart exercise and is good for you but not good for your body. If you are a female, please wear a jogging bra that is tight. You don't want your boobs lying on your belly when you are older. Power walking won't hurt your body, and you can get a very good workout, especially if you have hills in your area. You could also add some intermittent jog/walking. In my opinion, elliptical training machines are best for the least amount of stress to your body and getting the best heart workout but bounce your body and your face and are somewhat boring.

**Aerobics**

Dancing around to music is very fun but bouncing, as in running, is the dangerous part of this exercise. Injuries to knees, ankles, feet, hips, and arms are common. Low-impact aerobics are better.

**Spinning**

This is very hard on your knees. I only did a spinning class three times, and even though it was fun and hard work, it just wasn't right for my body or my knees.

After a workout session, if you are feeling pain in any joints or tissue, use the process of elimination to find out which exercise is hurting you. Look up stretches on the Internet. Stretching and rest is the only way to heal without surgery. If you have an injury and go to a surgeon, he will fix it with surgery. Try to heal yourself first by using rest, ice, and heat. Remember RICE; this acronym stands for:

**<u>R</u>est**
**<u>I</u>ce**
**<u>C</u>ompression**
**<u>E</u>levation**

Use ice for the first forty-eight hours, twenty minutes on and twenty minutes off, and then use moist heat after that.

Remember: Try to exercise without having it coming back to haunt you in your later years. If you are lucky, you will last into your later years with good health and with good bones and joints. The bottom line is, if it hurts, stop doing it and find another exercise.

Moderation is the key as you age. The combination of stretching, cardio, and lifting weights makes up true fitness. If you only do one component, you are not fit. You need each to be truly fit. If you can only do them two times per week, then do them two times per week; even once a week is better than none, but do them all.

I am currently working on a video of my stretching/yoga program. I have been doing these exercises for many years. They are not hard on your body and will allow you to remain flexible in your later years. I hope to be able to start filming this project soon!

*discipline is power*

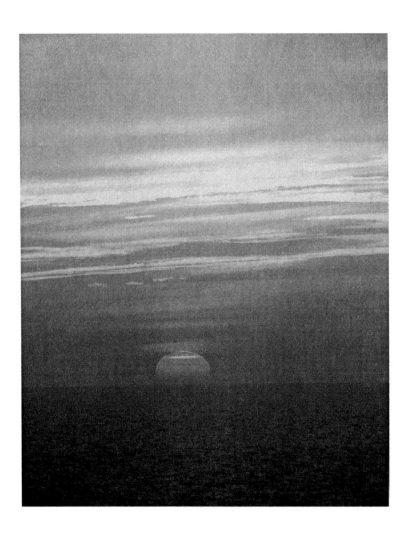

# chapter 11

# YOGA

*discipline is power*

༄

I was first introduced to yoga in the '90s at the fitness club where I worked. This was before my back surgery. I had a spinal fusion of L4 and L5 in 1998, after being in pain for twenty years. The lumbar vertebrae (lower area of the back) of the spinal column are defined by numbers going from one to five. I didn't want to have surgery, but, through the years, it just got to the point that the pain was unbearable, and I finally decided to have it fixed. Before surgery, I had trouble doing some of the Ashtanga (a form of yoga) poses, but I found a healthy backs class that helped slightly—not enough to avoid surgery, but it brought some relief.

After I got thrown out of the golf cart in 2007, I went to therapy and found that many of the stretches I was doing exacerbated the problem instead of helping. Now I have my own program that I do at home. In fact, my husband and I do it together. It takes about twenty minutes, three times a week, and it is wonderful. I hope to do a DVD to help other back pain sufferers. It gets rid of all the kinks in your neck, back, and hips. It also keeps us stretched out for golf and helps keep us strong.

My mantra is: DO NOT GO INTO OLD AGE UNLESS YOU ARE STRONG AND FLEXIBLE AND IN GOOD SHAPE. IT IS NOT FOR SISSIES. Actually it was my mother's mantra, and I stole it from her.

If you know nothing about stretching, start classes. Every neighborhood has yoga classes. Check with your neighbors and friends to see where they go. Most studios have online information. I would suggest starting out with a basic stretching program or beginner class, and after you feel that you are ready for a more strenuous class, go for it. You will feel better after you stretch every single time. I seriously don't understand how you can go through life not stretching. Everyone who doesn't stretch must have all kinds of aches and pains. I have none that can't be fixed by a session of stretching.

Every new golfer I play with always comments on my huge backswing and can't believe I have so much flexibility and torque. I don't think they mean at my age, either. I just think they don't see this kind of flexibility much on the golf course. It is because of my stretching program.

I used to sit with my mom at the retirement facility where she lived and everyone there had aches and pains. I would listen and always offer support and suggestions on how to help them. You, too, will feel better stretching a few times a week. **Flexibility is youth!**

*discipline is power*

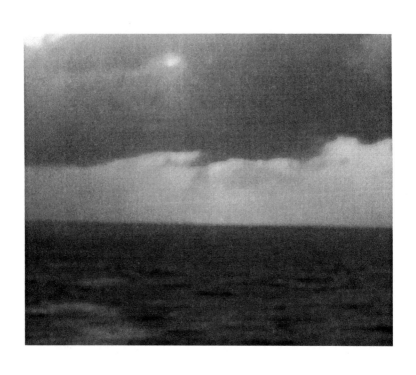

# chapter 12

# GETTING OFF SUGAR

*discipline is power*

༄

I told you in an earlier chapter that I would explain how to get off of sugar, and it is surprisingly simple. I was so addicted that I would wake up every morning and promise myself that I wasn't going to have chocolate or anything sweet that day, but by twelve o'clock in the afternoon, I had to go to the candy machine at work. I was obsessed by it. I could think of nothing else until I succumbed to the overwhelming desire. I would open the wrapper and take a bite, and all of a sudden I would get a rush, like I was putting a drug into my body. I could actually feel it going through me like a charge of electricity. I was a chocoholic and an addict. I would stop at the candy store on the way home from work. I was gaining weight so fast, I didn't know where to turn. I was panicking.

Luckily, we had a massage therapist at the club who was a holistic kind of guy. He was very memorable because, besides being so great looking, he couldn't keep his zipper up. He loved all the women, literally. He did more than massage his female clients. As I remember now, he was fired for just that. He did give me one of the tools to change my life, and I will never forget him. He was put in my path to save my life. Thank you, zipper boy!

The reason my body craved sugar so much was because I had recently quit smoking, and my heart rate, along with every other bodily function, dropped dramatically. I started smoking at the age of thirteen. I thought I was so cool then. Just remember, if you ever start smoking, sometime you will have to quit, and it is a very difficult and highly addictive habit to quit, so just **DON'T START**. We are already fighting disease every single day. What a dummy I was! I smoked for twenty-two years and am so thankful that I finally quit the fifth time.

The reason everyone always gains weight after quitting is because smoking is a stimulant and every time you take a puff, your bodily functions speed up and stay up. Think about it: Fifteen or twenty puffs on a cigarette, for a one-and-a-half-pack a day smoker, equals four hundred and fifty to six hundred puffs on a cigarette every day. My blood sugar and metabolism were pumped up by nicotine and chemicals constantly for twenty-two years. According to an article I read in the *Detroit Free Press* on the new e-cigarettes dated September 2, 2010, there are some 4,000 chemicals found in traditional cigarettes. I sucked the smoke into my body for all those years and didn't know the damage I was doing. Suddenly, when I quit, nothing was high anymore; everything dropped like a fifty-pound weight off a tall building.

But zipper boy, thankfully, was put in my path with the secret. He told me to take a bite, just a bite, of watery fruit every half-hour to stabilize my blood sugar. I used melon, oranges, grapes, anything watery, and I was shocked that if I followed his advice, my cravings disappeared. I was finally not addicted, and now, years later, indulge in sugar only at night and just a little.

In *The Fantastic Voyage*, Ray Kurzwell and Terry Grossman MD state that we did not evolve to consume the large quantities of refined sugars and starches that make up most of the modern diet. They are converted into sugar in the body almost immediately and produce carbohydrate (sugar) cravings. If you eat sugar in the morning, you will crave it all day. This means reading labels on cereal, oatmeal, and every other food you might be eating. Manufacturers sneak it into foods with names like high-fructose corn syrup, sucrose, and many other names. Look for sugar-free or low-sugar breads in the healthy foods or organic section of the grocery store.

When I followed zipper boy's advice, my weight stabilized, and I then began on a program of healthy eating and exercise for weight loss. It took me a while to get the weight off. I stopped weighing myself at one hundred and forty-five pounds and probably got close to one hundred and fifty pounds or more, which was a tremendous amount of weight for my petite five-two frame—but the time will go by anyway, so you might as well be doing something positive in the meantime!

Quitting sugar and smoking helped me begin to fight disease every day. I am sure you have read about these amazing people who have lost hundreds of pounds in a year or two. Just have patience, repeat your positive affirmations, and good things will happen for you. Know it, believe it, and say them out loud, so you can hear yourself in your mind talking about how you are changing your life for the better. **It's not what you achieve in life, but what you overcome.**

*discipline is power*

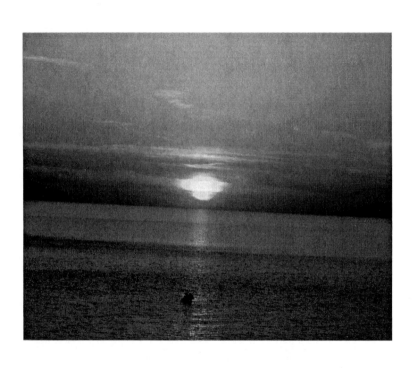

# chapter 13:

# SMOKING

*discipline is power*

෴

I feel that I am a pro at quitting smoking—I quit five times! A month here and month there. Two months here, two months there. Four times, I was sucked back in by taking one puff after my nicotine habit was gone.

According to Smoking Cessation, the class I took **twice** in 1979, given by the Seventh-Day Adventists, after a twenty-four-hour flush of fruit juice, the nicotine is flushed from your system. But one puff is all it ever took to suck me back in. I thought I could just have a puff every now and then. The truth is, if you have one puff after being addicted, you might just as well go buy a carton because within the next few days or weeks, you **will** be fully addicted again. That is how powerful cigarettes are. The secret to never smoking again after quitting is to never have that one puff ever again as long as you live.

With every urge, I always said to myself, "I will never have one puff again as long as I live." It works because you are telling your mind what you want, and it is listening. Quitting smoking is the most powerful tool you can have in your arsenal. When you finally quit, you feel that you can accomplish anything because you now have the power in yourself that cigarettes used to have over you. You take your life back, and you have the power. It is life changing, and I am very proud of myself and my many good friends who have also quit this very dangerous habit.

We didn't have nicotine drugs or patches back in the day like we do now. Cold turkey is the way I quit cigarettes, and if I did it, so can you. You kind of miss taking the stupid things everywhere you go, kind of like with your cell phone now.

Smoking wreaks havoc on your circulatory system and your heart. It ruins your beautiful skin that you want to look good until you're eighty or ninety. You sound like an old frog when you talk. Forget about doing anything athletic because you can't catch your breath. You have smoker's cough and are always coughing up crappy stuff from your lungs. My dental hygienist told me smoking melts your gums. No gums, no teeth. Last but not least, YOU STINK. Yes, you do. YOU STINK. If you kiss a nonsmoker, you will disgust them. One of my girlfriends still smokes and, as beautiful as she is, she can shower, put on her makeup, do her beautiful, long hair, and when I hug her hello, she stinks. Every single cigarette makes you sick.

I have two brothers who are five years apart, but people always ask which one is the older brother. Sorry, bro, but one of them is a one- or two-pack-a-day smoker and the other smokes a pack every two or three weeks. I could never figure out how he could smoke five to ten cigarettes a week, but he does it. The younger brother's skin is sallow in color and just doesn't look as healthy as the older one's. I have nagged him for years to quit. Thirty years ago I made him go to the dermatologist because of a black spot on his face that he never had before. He listened to me that time, and it turned out he had melanoma, a deadly form of skin cancer. They had to cut through six layers of his face to reach good cells. He could have died from that. Do you think he will listen to me about not smoking? Ha, no way.

The first time I quit smoking, I was twenty-one years old, and I tried to run around the block the day before I quit. I could only get two houses away. Can you imagine? At twenty-one years of age, I couldn't even run to the end of the street! The day I woke up and quit, I tried running again and ran halfway around the block before I got winded. Just one day later, my body started responding to pure oxygen instead of mixing chemicals with the air I needed to survive, and I was on the road to recovery. That was the first time—remember, I quit five times.

When I started smoking, cigarettes were only twenty-five cents a pack. I remember being on a cruise when I was sixteen and paying eighteen cents a pack. I think when I quit, they were up to sixty-five cents a pack. They are now over five dollars a pack, so if you only smoke one pack a day, you are wasting eighteen hundred and twenty-five dollars per year. If you smoke one and a half packs a day, you are wasting twenty-seven hundred and thirty-seven dollars per year. That is a lot of money that could go toward treating yourself to something really nice for quitting this awful habit.

If you want to stay healthy, quit smoking any way you can—pills, patches, or anything else that works—because it is the worst thing you can do to yourself. You have no idea how bad you smell if you smoke. Do your family and friends a favor: Quit smoking and start fighting disease right now.

*discipline is power*

# chapter 14:

# ALCOHOL

*discipline is power*

∽

Wine is mostly sugar. If you drink scotch or plain vodka, they are made with no added sugar. Wine has sugar left after the fermenting process, so if you are trying to get off the white stuff, stay away from wine and other sweet drinks. Add only club soda, water, or a wedge of lemon or lime to whiskey scotch or vodka. Scotch and vodka are eighty-six proof and have eighty-six calories in one ounce; one hundred-proof vodka has one hundred calories in one ounce. Bar pours are usually more. If you want to drink, make it a "low-sugar" alcoholic drink and just add it to your calorie allotment.

My nutritionist says all alcohol turns into sugar, but why add more by mixing your alcohol with sugary drinks? The experts say that one or two drinks a day is healthy, depending on your weight. Any amount over that and you are risking disease. Everything in moderation is a very good goal here.

I know very intimately the dangers of smoking and being an alcoholic. It is a deadly combination and even though you are getting self-gratification, if you develop cancer, your children are the ones who will suffer through the long months of chemo, the months of having a cancer-free diagnosis, and then the returning cancer. This cycle can continue over and over for years—then death. The years that cancer attacks are limitless and will strangle everyone close to you. It is a brutal disease, and you don't want to tempt fate when it comes to this very deadly illness. In Dr. Isadore Rosenfeld's book *Doctor, What Should I Eat*, he states that 3 percent of all cancers are caused by overuse of alcohol. Add smoking and you have a double whammy. The *national institutes of health Web site* states that the use of alcohol and smoking are among the factors that put people at risk for developing cancer. There are many good programs like Alcoholics Anonymous to help excessive drinkers. Seek them out in your area and go educate yourself. If you have a family member who is an alcoholic, try Al-anon meetings to help you and your children.

I had a friend who was a wonderful, smart, athletic, and intelligent girl, but she had a problem with alcohol. On many occasions, she got so wasted that I had to be a parent to her. After the fifth or sixth time, I had to break away from her because she was sucking the life out of me. Sometimes for your own health, you have to move along and leave friends behind. It's okay because you will find others to take their place, and they will find others to take yours. This life is about you and your happiness.

*discipline is power*

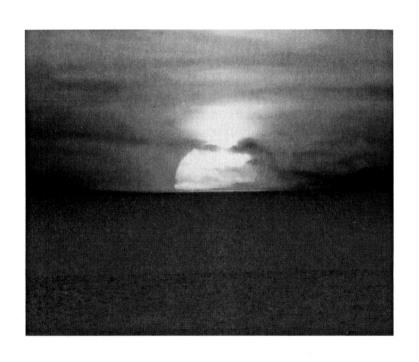

chapter 15:

# FAT

*discipline is power*

෧

We all see them, and they know who they are. The Center for Disease Control states that two out of three Americans are overweight. *Health Magazine,* May 2009, states that "sixty-five million American women are overweight or obese today and a new study predicts that in forty years all adults in the United States will be overweight or obese." This is crazy! Can you imagine the disease that will come with this prediction?

These are the people who fill the streets of every city and all our public places. Some people look at them with disgust; I have always looked at them with compassion, knowing that somewhere, down deep, they are tormented by something or someone, and I know they can be helped. No man or woman who is overweight is truly happy. If they say they are, they are lying. They just don't think they can be helped because their minds are so busy listening to all the negative things they have been saying for months or years and are therefore believing: "I can't lose weight," "I have been heavy for so long," "I am used to it," "It's in my genes," "I am big-boned," or "It's my thyroid condition."

You've seen them and, believe me, in my work, I have heard all the excuses.

I worked for a medical doctor after high school, and he knew how important weight was in relation to health. This was back in 1964. He was ahead of his time. He played handball every day on his lunch hour, so even back then he knew how important exercise was in relation to weight. He used to have sandbags in his office in increments of ten, twenty, fifty, and one hundred pounds. These were his tools to let his patients know how much extra weight their bodies were carrying around. He would make them lift and carry around the sand bags to really identify with the extra weight their bodies were forced to carry and lift every day. Have you ever tried to lift one hundred or even fifty pounds? I'll bet you can't do it. It's a lot easier if it's slapped onto your body or is it?

If you are a woman carrying fifty or one hundred extra pounds, your clothing is usually not very stylish, and you are probably a size twenty, twenty-two, or more; a man would wear a belt size of forty-eight or more. Your thighs rub together, and your belly is so big and hangs out so far that you can't see your shoes, which, by the way, are never comfortable. It is also very hard to get out of a chair or to bend over and pick something up off the floor. Often you are growing out of your clothes so quickly that they are too tight all the time. You would probably have several sizes of clothing in your closet. I always kept a pair of jeans that I wore when I was my thinnest before I gained my weight. I kept those jeans for fifteen years thinking that one day I would get back into them. I should have kept them twenty years, and I would have gotten into them. Ahh, what satisfaction that would have been.

Everyone carries their fat in different places. Sometimes you have belly fat, which experts say is the most dangerous because of danger to the heart. Sometimes you carry it in the thighs and hips, which is always unattractive, and, last but not least, sometimes in the butt. Some women have perfect symmetry and look good heavy but most don't. Fat can attack you anywhere you are genetically predisposed to carry it.

Internally, fat wraps itself around your major organs, wreaks havoc on your circulatory system, and, most importantly, engulfs your heart with fat. I will never forget the colored photograph of the human heart at a normal weight and the human heart overweight. I saw this amazing picture at the doctor's office where I worked. Picture the heart of a chicken or turkey with fat wrapped around it, like the greasy, disgusting stuff it is. That is what our heart looks like when we are overweight. How can it function normally?

My ex-mother-in-law, who is now deceased, carried three hundred and fifty pounds on her five-two frame for most of her adult life. She gained and lost hundreds of pounds in her lifetime. All she had to do was get off of sugar and starches to get to a healthy weight. She stayed many times at the Pauling Institute, a "fat farm" in Hyde Park, New York. She would fast for thirty days each time to cleanse her body, drinking only water. She would come home feeling terrific for a few weeks and was lighter by forty pounds or more. She felt skinny and terrific, even at three hundred pounds. But she gained all her weight back every time.

Her quality of life was so poor and got worse and worse as the years passed. She had bottles and bottles of pills. She had pills for high blood pressure, heart pills, water pills, gout pills, etc. She was so tired that she couldn't keep her house clean or walk to her car comfortably. She waddled when she walked and suffered so much for carrying that extra weight. She just sat on the couch with her potato chips by her side. They were her drug of choice. I never knew how to help her. She was obsessed with food and talked about it all the time. She was an addict. Starches turn into sugar in your system, and she was a heavy starch eater. As I sit here thinking about her, I realize she had no other interests: no community work, no reading, no volunteering, nothing—just TV and munching. But how can you do anything when you can't move around very well? Her whole life revolved around food.

Her husband was a saint and was very interested in keeping fit, which was so different than her. He was a very good-looking man, and he did everything for her. He cleaned and cooked and loved her very much. People would watch her in restaurants when she ate as if to say, "Why are you eating at your weight?" and, at the time, I am sorry to say, I was somewhat embarrassed by it. She found all her comfort in food and paid dearly for it. She had circulation problems, knee problems, hip problems, and foot problems. She was probably a diabetic, and I just never knew about it. She never made the commitment to try to look at weight from a health standpoint. I must say that we really didn't know what we know now about health and nutrition. It's pretty hard to be healthy when all you eat is fat, sugar, and starch.

The pictures of her as a young woman in her late teens were outstanding. She was stunning and slim, married her husband at sixteen, and, later, even at her tremendous weight, she was still beautiful. She died in a nursing home after many years in a wheelchair and lived much longer than I ever would have predicted. Maybe all the years of fasting on and off gave her body the cleansing that it needed. Her quality of life was very poor and extremely disturbing. Does this sound like anyone you know?

When I think of health insurance costs, I wonder why people who are fit, don't smoke, exercise regularly, and don't take drugs for chronic disease have to pay as much as someone who is obese, smokes, and doesn't exercise. The latter will face so many health problems over their lifetime. The insurance companies need to rethink their discount policies.

Some of the years I spent as sales manager at my club were the years when we were all trying to reduce the amount of fat in our diets. All the books came out about fat-free everything. After quitting smoking, I was at my all-time highest weight. It just kept going up, partly because my metabolism changed (after quitting smoking), and partly because I got the immediate addiction to sugar, which I spoke about earlier. I stopped weighing myself. I eliminated all the fat from my diet, hoping and praying to get skinnier. My diet allowed no meat or cheese and very little or no protein. I did eat lots of veggies and starch. Again, **starch turns into sugar in our bodies.**

During exercise, the body burns off the sugar (carbohydrates) first then the fat, so if you're eating a lot of starches and sugars, you will have to do an incredible amount of exercise to get to the stored fat. If the body has no carbohydrates to burn, it then goes after the stored fat, hence the high fat-low carbohydrate diets. I was exercising an hour a day, high-impact aerobics or running, eating fourteen hundred calories a day, and couldn't lose an ounce. The first time I remember having my cholesterol checked was sometime in 1992. I thought it would read around one hundred and seventy-five. Wrong! It was two hundred and forty-five. I thought I was doing everything right. I was eliminating the protein, which was fat, from my diet, but my blood work confirmed that I was doing everything wrong. The first cholesterol screening I tried to improve on was in August of 2001, at the age of fifty-four:

HDL 77—Good cholesterol. This number was always good because of exercise.
LDL 176—Bad cholesterol
Triglycerides 121
Total cholesterol 277
Ratio 3.6

My ratio, triglycerides, and HDLs were good, but everything else stunk. THE NUMBERS SHOULD BE:

HDL 45 or above
LDL 130 or below
Triglycerides 100-150
Total cholesterol 200 or less
Ratio 4.5 or below

Now, I was in heated competition with myself. I had to be better next time. I tried to get the numbers down by being even more diligent with my diet: mostly carbohydrates and no protein or fats. My next results were in January of 2002. Oh, horrors:

HDL 70
LDL 209
Triglycerides 134
Total cholesterol 306
Ratio 4.4

I was mortified. I couldn't believe it. I just couldn't get the numbers down. Two of my doctors wanted me to go on cholesterol medication. I told them I wanted to try some other things first. I wanted to become a total vegetarian to see if that would help.

Several years before this, I was diagnosed with osteoporosis. Thank you very much, low-fat diet! That was disappointing, and I had to start medication for osteoporosis immediately; I took it for seven years. I was very dedicated to being a vegetarian and told all my friends if we were going to dinner or if they were cooking for me, they would just have to understand that I was being a human guinea pig right then, so no meat, fish, poultry, or dairy. I was retested in July 2002, six months later. The results were encouraging but not as staggering as I had expected.

HDL 70
LDL 142
Triglycerides 163
Total cholesterol 245
Ratio 3.5

I had just about had it. Nothing I did could bring everything down to a point where I was comfortable with the numbers. It was then that I decided to try a modified Atkins diet. I remembered reading in his book about all the people who had their cholesterol levels come down and had other wonderful results from his diet. I started the diet in moderation. My weight by this time was under control only because I was highly active. I golfed several days a week and power walked four miles almost daily. I found that with the modified Atkins program, getting off of sugar and starch helped me maintain my weight for the first time in my life.

I was rechecked in May of 2003, ten months later:

HDL 100—I had always thought this number should be higher.
LDL 189
Triglycerides 36
Total cholesterol 296
Ratio 3.0

These numbers showed that you can have high total cholesterol, but in my opinion the ratio is what the real factor is. I am finally happy. Most doctors don't believe this, but as you read further, I will prove that, in my case, the ratio is the important number.

Even though some of the numbers went up, the important ones went down. My triglycerides went down from one hundred and sixty-three to thirty-five. That is a difference of one hundred and twenty-seven points. This is because the starches turn into sugar in your body, and since I was not eating much of either sugar or starch, the high sugar content in my body was much lower. My HDL (healthy cholesterol) went from seventy up to one hundred. That is thirty points better. I don't believe I did anything different as far as exercise to make this happen. The ratio went down .05 percent. This is good— really good. My doctors were surprised. They had been telling me all along to exercise more, do weight-bearing exercises, and cut out the cholesterol in my foods. I kept telling them I did all that, so it was just very confusing.

It took me a few years to figure it out, but I am happy. I am sticking with what works. I am passing this information on to you so that you can benefit from me, the human guinea pig.

The final confirmation came when friends of ours had heart scans a few years later and told us about this incredible test. At that time, it was a new test, paid for out-of-pocket and pretty expensive, but it was money well spent.

My husband and I made the appointment and went off to our heart scans. The test confirmed, surprisingly, that I had absolutely no plaque buildup. Understand:

zero and didn't need medication for my cholesterol. The doctors were wrong! Now, I was really happy.

My husband, who has always had low cholesterol of around one hundred and seventy-five and a resting heart rate of fifty-two, had a 10 to 15 percent plaque buildup. Go figure! I found out the reason why years later in my research.

I have been reading and trusting Dr. Mercola, who is a DO, a *Times* best-selling author, and an osteopathic physician. Osteopathic physicians' approach toward medicine is more holistic, and they treat the entire person rather than a collection of symptoms. They also help patients develop attitudes and lifestyles that don't just fight illness but work on prevention, too. I like his style and read his column regularly. After looking into his education, I realized I like him more than ever. His education is as follows:

University of Illinois at Urbana-Champaign, 1972-1976

Chicago College of Osteopathic Medicine, 1978-1982

Chicago Osteopathic Hospital, 1982-1985, Family Practice Residency. Chief resident, 1984- 1985

Board Certified American College Osteopathic General Practitioners, July 1985

State of Illinois Licensed Physician and Surgeon

According to Dr. Mercola in his January 26, 2010, e-mail, the new research of why this happened to me was: There are two types of LDL—and only one is bad!

In the 1970s, low-density lipoproteins (LDLs) were discovered. LDLs were found to be higher in people with cardiovascular disease, so the focus of medicine and nutrition became lowering your LDLs. One of the crucial pieces of the puzzle that wasn't recognized at the time was that *there are two kinds of LDL: Pattern A and Pattern B.*

1. Pattern A LDLs are large, light, buoyant "floating" LDLs that don't get under your endothelial cells, and they don't cause plaque formation. They are harmless.
2. Pattern B LDLs (or VLDLs) are smaller, denser LDLs that are able to wedge themselves under your epithelial cells and therefore roughen surfaces and stimulate plaque formation. *These are the bad guys.*

Unfortunately, when you get a standard lipid profile at your annual checkup, the LDL measured is a combination of both types. Lab measurements lump them together unless you have a very specialized panel, which most physicians don't order.

To decipher whether or not you have an excess of the bad type, you can look at your triglycerides and high-density lipoprotein (HDL) levels. (HDL, or high density lipoprotein is commonly called "good cholesterol.")

Here is a simple way to determine if you have too much bad LDL:

1. If your triglycerides are low and your HDL is high, then the LDL you have is the good variety.

2. If your triglycerides are high and your HDL is low, then the LDL you have is the bad variety. **The triglyceride-to-HDL ratio is a far better indicator of cardiovascular disease** than the total cholesterol-to-HDL ratio **that** everyone uses.

Now, here's the bottom line: Dietary fat raises your large, buoyant LDL—the one that is harmless. **Dietary sugar raises your small, dense LDL—the one that correlates with heart disease!** Hurray for Dr. Mercola because, for years, I wondered how this could happen.

Another interesting thing happened when I received my most recent blood work, and my platelet count was three hundred and seven. Normal is one hundred and forty-five to three hundred and fifty-five. Upon **investigation on the Web, I found that the higher the number (even though this is not high, it is higher than average) it means** increased platelet counts may be seen in individuals who show no significant medical problems,. Some, although they have an increased number of platelets, may have a tendency to bleed due to *the lack of stickiness* of the platelets; in others, the platelets retain their stickiness but, because they are increased in number, they tend to stick to each other, forming clumps that can block a blood vessel and cause damage, including death. I like knowing that my blood is not sticking together to form clots or blockages. I believe this paragraph explains why I tend to get bluish-purplish bruises occasionally on my forearms.

Last week I was at a function and met a very nice young woman. I asked her what she did and she replied that she was a nurse practitioner. I love meeting these types of people because I always pick their brains. I wanted to know the difference between a nurse practitioner and a physician's assistant. She told me that she could hang a shingle and the physician's assistant would have to work under the physician.

I asked her about the Pattern A and Pattern B cholesterol and she told me that I would have to ask for a test called lipoprotein A. They wouldn't do the test without my asking. This would confirm whether I had Pattern A or Pattern B cholesterol. Neither of my doctors who wanted me on cholesterol medication offered or suggested this test to me. I had to find out in a social function from a woman off the street. Thank you, Ms. Nurse Practitioner, for your information and taking the time to answer all my questions.

Five years later, I heard this inner voice that said we should go get another heart scan just to follow up. I wanted to confirm that my husband didn't have any additional blockage. I love my husband and want to keep him around for a long time, so I called to set up the appointment. They offered us a body scan, which was kind of new at the time, a little more expensive, and not covered by insurance, but I figured again it was money well spent. I made the appointment for the body scans and thought it was no big deal.

That night, they called and said I was fine but my husband had kidney cancer. We were in shock! How could we tell our children? My heart goes out to all who have had a cancer diagnosis; it is the scariest thing ever. We were hit with a blow that we never expected. We walked around in a fog for three months. We waited as long as we could and told our kids just before he had his biopsy. They were all there for the surgery.

My husband had always watched his diet and exercised regularly, so we thought he was very healthy. He had parents who lived a long life into their nineties without disease. How could he have cancer? Luckily, he was diagnosed at stage one, which is almost unheard of unless someone is going through another health issue, and it is caught by mistake—or unless you are smart enough to have a body scan. His life was saved by this amazing test. No chemo and very little recovery after his partial nephrectomy.

Three years later, he is cancer free and wears a Live Strong bracelet, which is meant to unite people to fight cancer, believing that unity is strength, knowledge is power, and attitude is everything! Lance Armstrong, a well-known athlete and survivor of testicular cancer, created these bracelets.

I believe strongly in being proactive regarding your health and tell my husband he always has to be nice to me because I saved his life!

*discipline is power*

# chapter 16:

# THYROID CONDITIONS

*discipline is power*

∽

Upon investigation on the Internet, I learned that the thyroid is one of the largest endocrine glands in the body. It is found in the neck and controls how quickly the body uses energy, makes proteins, and controls how sensitive the body should be to other hormones.

The thyroid participates in these processes by producing thyroid hormones, principally thyroxine ($T_4$) and triiodothyronine ($T_3$). These hormones regulate the rate of metabolism and affect the growth and rate of function of many other systems in the body. Iodine and tyrosine are used to form both $T_3$ and $T_4$. The thyroid also produces the hormone calcitonin, which plays a role in calcium homeostasis. Calcium homeostasis means how the body governs calcium levels. The thyroid is monitored by the hypothalamus and pituitary glands.

That description is all too technical for me, but I know that it is a very important part of good health. My nutritionist, Dr. Guiterrez, recently told me that 95 percent of the nation's population has thyroid disease. Do you realize how many of us have this issue? When I walked into his office, he diagnosed me immediately. As it turns out, after taking my temperature each morning for a week under my arm just as I opened my eyes, sure enough, my temperature ranged from 95.5 to 96.7. Normal should be 98.6. Hypothyroidism is the proper term. It means an underactive thyroid.

I am now taking iodine, which is a natural, holistic treatment. My blood pressure has also been very low for my entire life. It would range between 107/72 and 112/73, but now I am 120/80, which is within the range of perfect blood pressure. This was an unexpected surprise of taking iodine.

During my research, I found that the thyroid also controls your calcium levels. I am thinking that this may be a contributing factor as to why my calcium levels have been so low for years and the calcium medication I was on for seven years never helped. We will find out after my next bone density test.

Symptoms of hypothyroidism are:
- Dry, thinning hair
- Depression
- Poor memory
- Tiredness and lethargy
- Swollen face, hands, and feet
- Muscle pain
- Joint pain
- Dry skin
- Sensitivity to cold
- Brittle, thin fingernails
- Constipation
- Weight gain
- Slower movements and speech

Less common symptoms include:
- Thickening of facial features
- Thinning eyebrows
- Reduced sense of taste and smell
- Hoarseness or deepening of the voice
- Slow heart rate
- Heavier periods
- Fertility problems
- Increased risk of miscarriage
- Decreased libido

According to Dr. Oz, another symptom of low thyroid could be the last half of one's eyebrow disappearing. Also high LDLs when you eat healthy. One of my daughters had classic symptoms for at least fifteen years and none of her many doctors diagnosed her. She is very smart and knew she had a thyroid condition, but her tests never showed it. She would find a new doctor every year or two, get retested, and was never diagnosed. We think it is because when you order a thyroid test there has to be three levels of testing; this is the proper way to diagnose thyroid disease. You must get the TSH thyroid-stimulating test. Thanks to Dr. Guiterrez, she had the proper testing done and guess what? She needed thyroid medication. Finally, she is starting to feel healthy and energetic.

A very good friend of mine has a daughter who started having problems with depression in her late teens and early twenties. Of course, the doctor prescribed antidepressants for her immediately. I am not sure if they did any blood tests at all on her, but he immediately got out the prescription pad and started her on a fifteen-year battle with medication. Before long, she was taking sleep aids and different kinds of very strong medication because, once you start with a medication, there is always a side effect and then there is another medication to stop the side effects of that medication, and then you get side effects from that medication, and on and on and on. Before you know it, you are on five or more medications a day, and you still don't feel better. Recently, there was an extremely low point for this girl, and she entered a hospital for detoxification. After speaking to my friend, I suggested that she could be suffering from hypothyroidism. Her weight was up to one hundred and ninety pounds, and she had every single symptom of this disease. I was so thankful that I chose to call her that day because now if she has a thyroid condition they can begin to treat her properly. This is a bright and talented girl, but because of not being aware of certain things, she and her family have suffered through all of her depression problems her whole adult life.

Another good friend and I were speaking recently and she shared with me that she just wasn't feeling like herself lately; she had been feeling very tired, her hair was thinning, and she had other related issues. She was also going through menopause. She was beside herself with confusion as to why she was feeling like this after so many years of feeling great. Sounded like a thyroid condition to me, so I immediately suggested that maybe this would be something that she should get tested for. She then said to me, "I have been taking thyroid medication for twenty-five years." Being a layperson, but with good common sense, it seems to me that since all our hormones go through incredible changes during menopause, thyroid hormone levels should change right along with estrogen and progesterone levels. So if you are feeling like my friend, get tested or retested. She is getting tested, and I am sure her levels are different than they were before.

I recently spoke to another friend who shared with me her difficulty in getting pregnant for three years after her marriage. She went to an infertility doctor who immediately put her on synthroid (a thyroid medication) and after one month of being on the drug, she got pregnant; she had two subsequent pregnancies. She has been on synthroid for twenty-two years.

There is also the condition of having an overactive thyroid. The symptoms of hyperthyroidism tend to reflect the rapid metabolism that results from an oversupply of thyroid hormones. Common symptoms include:

- Anxiety
- Rapid weight loss
- Diarrhea
- High heart rate
- High blood pressure
- Eye sensitivity/bulging
- Vision disturbances
- Insomnia

A properly working thyroid is a very complex but vitally important part of our well-being. If you are having any of these symptoms, please see a health care professional armed with this essential information. During my research, I found that low thyroid is also linked to low calcium levels, so I am hoping that the iodine I am taking will help my calcium levels. I am absolutely certain it will.

*discipline is power*

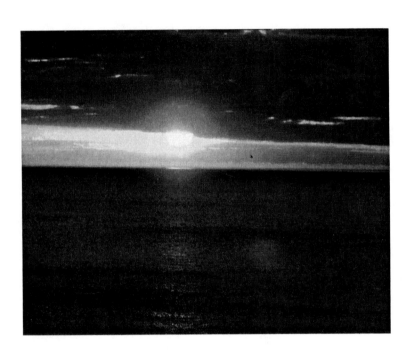

# chapter 17

# OSTEOPOROSIS

*discipline is power*

∽

I was taking six calcium supplements per day, plus taking Actonel, a prescription bone loss regimen, regularly for osteoporosis, but I still kept losing bone mass. How could that be?

For seven years, I was on a fat-free program and eating very small amounts of protein. This is what the "experts" said to do to lose and maintain weight. A few months before my yearly checkup, I stopped taking all of it. It was around the same time that I was on the modified Atkins program. I went drug free for four months and occasionally would think of myself at eighty all bent over but quickly dismissed it. No Actonel, no calcium, nothing. It was great being free from taking any drugs.

To my unbelievable surprise, at my next appointment, I no longer had osteoporosis. I was better. I was diagnosed with osteopenia, which is a preosteoporosis condition. Even the prescription medication I took for seven years never helped me gain bone. Now I was really surprised because I never, ever thought that the modified Atkins would help my osteoporosis.

I am now drug free and love it! At the age of sixty-four, I am still in osteopenia, which is good for me since I am a petite woman and osteoporosis usually strikes women who have a slight build. I directly relate the added bone mass to the protein, the modified Atkins way of eating, and the iodine supplements. I try to stick with his program by adding more healthy carbohydrates, and have only a little sugar and only at night.

Too bad Dr. Atkins got such a bad rap. In my opinion, he was way ahead of his time and was a genius.

*discipline is power*

# chapter 18

# GENES

*discipline is power*

∽

Just for example, my family's genes are very interesting.

My dad—the loving, wonderful man that he was—died at seventy-three of heart disease. He never exercised, loved sugar, was thirty-five pounds or more overweight, smoked on and off for thirty years, and made the commitment to change his life too late. His sister exercised regularly, never smoked, and died at ninety-eight. She had Alzheimer's and couldn't remember me at ninety-three or ninety-four. She was an avid exerciser who went to body recall classes three times a week her whole adult life. For as long as I can remember, she went on fast, long walks and was always interested in keeping fit. Unfortunately, she forgot about her mind. Experts say that it is very important to keep learning and growing in your mind as you grow older. Boy, was she ahead of her time with her exercise program. Maybe some of her lifestyle choices rubbed off on me, and I never knew it.

Their brother, my Uncle Ed, is an amazing man. He is so cute, living in the independent living area where there are over five hundred residents. He is the resident stud. The women love him and so do I. He is a retired colonel from the United States Air Force and was active in WWII. He was a fighter pilot, and at his age of ninety-four, he still walks like a military man. He also exercises regularly. He played racquetball until he was into his nineties and weight trains, does the treadmill, plays water polo, and plays Ping-Pong now. He is computer literate and very, very smart. If you saw him walking from behind, you would think he was a man in his forties or fifties. He is one of my mentors, as was his sister.

It seems to me that if my father exercised and watched his lifestyle like his brother and sister, he may have lived to meet my husband. My greatest disappointment in life is that they never met. Now that I think about it, their mother, my grandmother, always walked everywhere she went. I don't remember her having a car, ever. She always exercised, even in her apartment; she would walk up and down the steps from the first floor to the second floor ten times, twice a day, and always did toe touches. She lived to be ninety three.

My husband's family is also interesting. All four of his grandparents cleared ninety and one lived to be a hundred years old. They were born and raised in Czechoslovakia and Italy and came to live in the United States as young adults. They were not exposed to junk food or fast food and lived a long and healthy life. His parents both lived into their nineties and had lots of Italian food, wine, and no fast food or junk food. She prepared everything they ate. His father never went to the doctor until he was in his late eighties. His mother had every joint replacement that you could have—hips, knees, aortic valve replacement, pacemaker—but no health-related problems such as cancer or tumors. Dad lived to ninety-two and Mom lived to ninety-four.

These generations were just like ours except we are supposed to be smarter about nutrition and lifestyles today. We have done the research so we should know. Fast food, processed foods, junk food, sugar, corn oil, butter, cigarettes, cigars, overuse of alcohol, and lack of exercise are the reasons we have health issues in our fifties and sixties. We get heart problems from smoking and lack of exercise, and liver issues from drinking too much alcohol. One of the worst problems is obesity from overindulging in empty calories containing starches and sugar.

Genes are a big issue, but if you take care of yourself, your chances of living longer are better than your parents'.

*discipline is power*

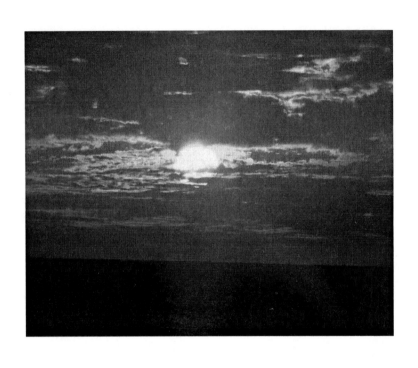

chapter 19:

# DIABETES

*discipline is power*

༄

Diabetes is deadly. It is a ravaging disease that kills body parts one at a time. I am a volunteer at a local hospital, and in the fifteen years that I have been doing this, I have seen cases where diabetes has taken toes, feet, fingers, and limbs.

Type II diabetes can be controlled by diet. Keep your weight in control as you age or your risk of developing this disease is elevated. There are two types of diabetes, but both are deadly if undiagnosed.

At first, your blood sugar level may rise so slowly that you may not know that anything is wrong. In fact, one-third of all people who have diabetes do not know they have the disease.

According to *About.com,* symptoms of Type I diabetes usually develop quickly, over a few days to weeks, and are caused by blood sugar levels rising above the normal range (hyperglycemia). Early symptoms may be overlooked, especially if the person has recently had an illness, such as the flu. Early symptoms include:

- Frequent urination, which may be more noticeable at night. Some young children who have learned

to use the toilet may start wetting the bed during
naps or at night.
- Extreme thirst and a dry mouth
- Weight loss
- Increased hunger (possibly)

Sometimes the blood sugar level rises excessively
before a person knows something is wrong. Because
insulin is not available, the cells in the body are unable
to get the sugar (glucose) they need for energy. The
body begins to break down fat and muscle for energy.
When fat is used for energy, ketones, or fatty acids,
are produced and enter the bloodstream, causing the
chemical imbalance of diabetic ketoacedosis. This is
a life-threatening condition. Symptoms of diabetic
ketoacidosis are:

- Flushed, hot, dry skin
- Loss of appetite, abdominal pain, and vomiting
- A strong, fruity breath odor
- Rapid, deep breathing
- Restlessness, drowsiness, difficulty waking up,
  confusion, or coma. Young children may lack
  interest in their normal activities.

Symptoms of Type II diabetes may include:
- Feeling thirsty
- Having to urinate more than usual
- Feeling hungrier than usual
- Losing weight without trying to
- Feeling very tired
- Feeling cranky

Other signs of Type II diabetes may include:
- Infections, cuts, and bruises that heal slowly
- Blurred vision
- Tingling or numbness in your hands or feet
- Trouble with skin, gum, or bladder infections
- Vaginal yeast infections

Get your child or yourself to a health care professional immediately if you have any of these symptoms.

*discipline is power*

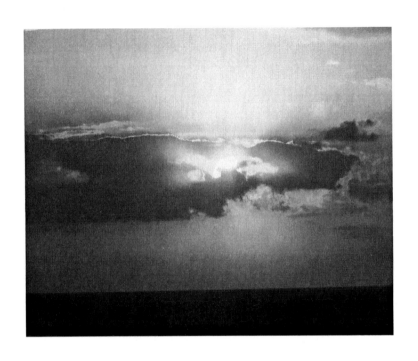

# chapter 20

# THERMOGRAPHY OR MAMMOGRAPHY

*discipline is power*

∽

A few years ago, it was brought to my attention by a casual friend that there was an alternative to mammography that was safer and easier, and could detect breast cancer eight years before conventional mammography. It is thermography.

Thermography images are captured in real time from an ultrasensitive medical infrared imaging camera and sent to a sophisticated computer for storage and analysis (the images are kept on a computer for precision comparison of future images so that the breasts can be monitored over time). Sophisticated computer programs allow the doctor to isolate temperature differentials, perform analyses and studies. Dr. William Cockburn stated in 2002 in his article about thermography that breast thermography is very accurate.

I never cared much for mammography testing and often thought since I had no breast cancer in my family, mammograms were not necessary every year. Also, being within a normal weight range, I would not be a strong candidate for breast cancer. It also bothered me that I had to have a prescription from my doctor before they would test me. I really don't understand what the thinking is. It seems that I should just be able to take my insurance card at age thirty and get a mammogram on my own.

That said, I still had them every year for about ten years and then every two years from my mid-fifties on. I had decided that I was not going to have mammograms again and just have thermograms until I met a radiologist at my brother's wedding who nixed my thinking about that. He is a radiologist, and they make their money reading X-rays. Besides that, hospitals have invested an incredible amount of money in their diagnostic machines, so, after meeting him, he talked me into another mammogram. I made my appointment upon return, but I also had the thermogram. I have been having thermograms for about three or four years; they are easy, quick, and one hundred and fifty dollars out of pocket.

When my husband had cancer of the kidney, it was encapsulate and stage one. According to my nutritionist, when it is encapsulated, it means it is in a protective, healthy layer so that it won't break open, allowing cancer to spread to other cells or organs. Stage one means just the beginning stage of cancer; stage four is the worst. His body was doing what it was supposed to do. If, by chance, you have breast cancer, and your body is doing what it is supposed to do by encapsulating the cancer, but you have a mammogram, and they squash your breast like a sandwich on a panini maker. What is going to happen to that breast cancer that is just lying there in a dormant, protective stage? Will it break open and spread? I don't know, but it does make me question mammograms.

Our urologist, Dr. J. Stuart Wolf, at the University of Michigan Hospital, told us that some doctors believe that even if you have a biopsy or surgery on a cancer site, your cancer could spread quickly because the protective barrier, the encapsulation, is broken between the cancer and your body. He didn't believe that to be the case.

Regular diagnostic mammograms expose you to low levels of radiation. In her book *Life's Delicate Balance*, Janette D. Sherman, MD states that X-rays are the most commonly known form of man-made radiation energy exposure and continual radiation is cumulative. This is the reason women in their twenties and thirties are not advised to have mammograms. David E. Goldberg, PhD, Chief of Genetic Epidemiology Group at the International Agency for Research on Cancer in Lyon, France, advises breast MRIs for these women. Talk about cancer-causing substances—could this be one of the reasons we have so much breast cancer today? How about the false positives? I had to go back for another mammogram and more radiation for a false positive at one point. If I had to go back, think of all the other women who have to go back. So my decision is not to have any more mammograms. I will have thermograms every year or maybe every six months for prevention. You have to make your own decision by being an informed patient.

Where I work as a volunteer at my local hospital, I just received their spring 2010 health letter, where there was an article about mammography versus thermography. It states:

If you are at a higher risk of cancer, your physician can recommend a breast MRI in addition to a screening mammogram or instead of a mammogram. Not every imaging center offers breast MRI, and the American Cancer Society recommends choosing a facility that also offers MRI-guided breast biopsy to avoid having the test repeated when the biopsy is done.

I question whether a mammogram is the best choice. If you are going to be a patient, question your doctor; ask lots of questions so you get all the answers you want. Doctors are not gods, even though I have met some who think they are.

About seven or eight years ago, I went to a doctor's appointment with my mother. I asked one question and this female doctor acted like I couldn't be smart enough to question her decision, as if I shouldn't have even been there to question anything she said or did because everything she did was right. I think, in some cases, doctors *practice* medicine because they are not absolutely sure of anything. She barked at me for questioning her and, plainly, she was a stone-cold bitch, so she lost my mother as a patient immediately. I loved my mom and wanted the best care for her. I am an informed woman who questions everything, and I want answers to my questions without attitude.

I recently read in an article in *Experience Magazine*, May 2010, that "one of the most overlooked keys to happiness is cultivating and exercising our innate sense of curiosity. That's because it creates openness to unfamiliar experiences, laying the groundwork for greater opportunities to experience discovery, joy, and delight." Works for me, considering I question everything! If a doctor doesn't have time or seems put off by your questions, find another doctor because you need one with compassion, especially if you are going through some sort of health issue.

I recently golfed with a woman who shared a story with me that I have to pass along. She was in her mid-fifties and went through a horrendous experience after being diagnosed with breast cancer. When she told me that she was a breast cancer survivor, I asked her if she wouldn't mind if I asked her questions about it. (I told you I ask questions about everything. Sometimes I drive my husband crazy!) She said not at all, and during our four-hour round of golf, she informed me of things that no woman in this day and age should ever have to go through.

She went to have her yearly mammogram and the radiologist said she should come back in six months since they found something questionable, but everything would be fine until reexamination. When this happened to me, I was scared to death. When I went for my retest, they said they could give me my results immediately. I was not prepared to have the results that quickly, but I turned out to be just fine. Three days after this woman's mammogram, her very good friend, who was a doctor, called her and said they needed a guinea pig for a new machine they were testing. It was a breast MRI.

Magnetic resonance imaging (MRI) is a noninvasive medical test that helps physicians diagnose and treat medical conditions. MRI imaging uses a powerful magnetic field, radio frequency pulses, and a computer to produce detailed pictures of organs, soft tissues, bone, and virtually all other internal body structures.

The images can then be examined on a computer monitor, transmitted electronically, and printed or copied to a CD. MRI does not use ionizing radiation (X-rays). Detailed MRI images allow physicians to better evaluate various parts of the body and determine the presence of certain diseases that may not be assessed adequately with other imaging methods, such as X-rays, ultrasound, or computed tomography (also called CT or CAT scanning). MRI of the breast offers valuable information about many breast conditions that cannot be obtained by other imaging modalities, such as mammography or ultrasound. (This is the test I would want if I were getting my breasts examined. I believe this test is very expensive and not many locations are available, so insurance companies would rather their clients have traditional testing.)

So, this woman complied with her friend's wishes and went to her appointment the next day. Remember, this was three days after her mammogram. During the test, her doctor friend and the technician were looking at the images and all of a sudden they said, "Oh, this does not look good. I don't like the looks of that." The next minute they were telling her that she had a very aggressive form of breast cancer and needed immediate treatment. God bless her friend.

She immediately made appointments at some high-profile hospitals to decide where to go for treatment. She saw three very well-known doctors in three different cities. Each one came in to speak to her about treatment and talked about her breasts like they were not even in the same room, let alone part of her body. They were all very condescending and not compassionate. Here was this lovely woman who had just been hit with the blow of her life, and she couldn't get one of the three doctors to show a hint of remorse for her. One doctor even said to her, "Well, we could take off one or we could take off two. It's up to you," without giving her any hint of compassion or statistics. She was even more devastated.

She finally found the fourth doctor, whom she very much loved, and decided to have a double mastectomy. With her first drop of chemo treatment, she blacked out after a fire of pain went through her body. It turned out that she was allergic to that type of chemo, and it almost killed her. Don't you think that after all the research money donated to breast cancer, they would know to test someone first to see if they were allergic to that type of chemo?

This woman is healthy and alive today in spite of the mammogram and the three idiot doctors. She also has breast implants perfect for her size. Not a bad golfer, either.

With every question comes a learning experience. I doubt that her mammogram released her aggressive breast cancer, but I don't know that it didn't. All I *do* know is that you have to be well informed to be able to make a decision that is right for you.

I question that with all the money donated to cancer research that in thirty years there has been nothing to replace mammograms as the protocol for diagnosing breast cancer.

*discipline is power*

# chapter 21

# HORMONES AND OTHER DRUGS

*discipline is power*

❧

Hormones, in my opinion, do more harm than good. My advice is DO NOT TAKE THEM. After I read *What Your Doctor May Not Tell You About Menopause*, by Dr. John R. Lee, with Virginia Hopkins, I was shocked. The book is primarily about hormones and hormone replacement therapy. The whole world was put on them after a dubious study on a small number of women already taking birth control pills in Puerto Rico. It was a carefully calculated media campaign of greed. This is how they got the approval as a prescription drug. They put the whole civilized world on them for years, and it was only after women started getting uterine and breast cancer that the link was found between HRT and cancers.

As far as HRT is concerned, go through your menopause and hot flashes with a hand fan and layer your clothing. For some women, hot flashes only last a few years; for others, much longer. Layer your clothing down to a summer sleeveless shirt in the winter months, so you can strip your clothes down to a spaghetti strap top for immediate relief when you have a hot flash.

I **do not** recommend soy supplements. After not having a period for a year, they made me start again after taking them for only six months. My gynecologist recommended a DNC—dilation and curettage. It is a procedure where they dilate your cervix and scrape your uterus with a spoon-shaped instrument. I was shocked at how hard recovering from this surgical procedure was. I was down and out for over a week. It was the worst recovery I ever had to have. I think the DNC was worse than the spinal fusion I went through. Men shouldn't use soy products as they mimic estrogen, a female hormone and may affect erections.

Let your body do what it is supposed to do. It is a wonderful thing not to have periods anymore, so try to think positively about the end result. Carry a hand fan in your purse and keep the room cold when you sleep. Sleep in short, light nightgowns or naked, and you will get through it.

I don't trust drug companies nor do I trust their test results. Greed is everywhere. The doctors only know what the pharmaceutical salespeople and the periodicals tell them. Have you ever seen so many advertisements for Viagra and Cialis? They would have you believe that the whole world is having erection problems!

The following are some examples of problems with drug testing. In a recent newsletter, I read that Dana Ullman, who is an author of ten books on homeopathic medicine, wrote:

> "There are many physicians who do not see
> there is something fundamentally wrong with

the present medical model...For the majority of people facing chronic illness, drugs provide short-term results, serious side effects, and the stratospherically high costs benefit the drug companies. Across the board, pharmaceutical companies do an excellent job of publicizing the findings they want you to know, while keeping quiet about the rest."

One of the things that have come out recently about some of the antidepressant research is how many studies had negative results, but they are almost never published. Only the ones with the positive results are published and, according to the FDA, drug companies only need to have two positive studies, which is enough for acceptance. In my opinion, that is a serious problem because if you keep trying, the law of averages will come up with something positive.

Even published studies can be seriously flawed. In her book *The Truth about Drug Companies: How They Deceive Us and What to Do About It*, Dr. Marcia Angell, who was the former editor in chief of the *New England Journal of Medicine*, stated that she exposed many examples of why medical studies often cannot be trusted. She stated that:

"Trials can be rigged in a dozen ways, and it happens all the time. For instance, most medical studies only examine a drug's effect in isolation and for a very short period of time. Its claims of efficacy or safety are therefore null and void if a person intends to take a drug for a longer period or in combination with other drugs, but this faux pas is ignored by the medical community."

The average American is not taking just one drug. They are often on many drugs and people need to know that there simply is very, very little science—often no science—behind the use of multiple drugs used concurrently. Most of the science that has been done is with one drug at a time and, in fact, with many of the psychiatric medications, they have only been tested for a small amount of time.

Most research claims cannot be trusted. Back in 2005, Dr. John Ioannidis, an epidemiologist at Ioannina School of Medicine in Greece, showed that there is "less than a 50 percent chance that the results of any randomly chosen scientific paper will be true." Then, in 2008, Dr. Ioannidis again showed that much of "scientific research being published is highly questionable." According to his study, "Simulations show that for most study designs and settings, it is more likely for a research claim to be false than true."

He noted problems with experimental and statistical methods as the main culprits, including factors such as small sample sizes, poor study design, researcher bias, and selective reporting. Because of the way the system runs, journals may be more likely to publish studies that show dramatic results, positive results, or results from "hot" competitive fields. For instance, a Cochrane Collaboration review and analysis of published flu vaccine studies found that flu vaccine studies sponsored by industry are treated more favorably by medical journals even when the studies are of poor quality.

Most "scientific" solutions also cover up symptoms. The drug-based solutions that medical research intends to "prove" are flawed by their very nature. They are solutions that simply cover up symptoms and do nothing to address the cause of the problem; in fact, they may actually harm you.

A good friend of mine recently died of brain cancer shortly after he was diagnosed with esophageal cancer. I spoke to his son recently, and he told me that his father's heartburn was so intense as a young man that he remembers him standing on his head for relief. Pretty extreme, but if you are in that much pain, you will do anything for relief. He also said that the doctor told his family that even if you take medication to cure the pain of constant heartburn, the medication only masks the symptoms; the heartburn is still there. The doctor and the family believe that constant heartburn led to his esophageal cancer. If you have constant heartburn, try to find out what causes it and stay away from that food item. My ex-husband had heartburn for years, and it was caused by coffee; he knew it and chose not to give it up, so he suffered every day.

Another example of problems with medication is Accutane, a drug that was recently pulled off the market in 2009. Hoffman LaRoche discontinued the manufacture of Accutane citing dwindling market share because of generics, however, there were many lost claims against them.

After losing a $33 million lawsuit in June of 2009, Roche Pharmaceuticals pulled Accutane off the U.S. markets. Approximately 13 million people have taken Accutane since it was introduced in 1982, and there are numerous lawsuits against Roche that are still pending because of claims of bowel disease.

In November of 2008, three Accutane users were awarded $12.9 million by an Atlantic City, New Jersey, jury because of claims that the drug caused long-term IBD (inflammatory bowel disease). A total of almost $21 million was awarded in three separate lawsuits in New Jersey and Florida because of cases involving Accutane causing long-term IBD.

I have a friend whose son was in critical condition, lost thirty-five pounds, and was in and out of the hospital for the last several months trying to get back to good health, all thanks to taking Accutane when he was in his early teens. Thirteen million people, many of them young children, have had problems with this drug. Almost thirty years later, the drug companies say, "Oh, sorry...we made a mistake."

On May 25, 2010, in the *Detroit Free Press*, it was reported that a subsidiary of Johnson and Johnson was accused of illegally promoting Topamax, a medicine only approved for seizures and migraine headaches. They were promoting it for other uses, including obesity in children without epilepsy, as well as mood disorders and alcohol dependence in adults. This drug was promoted by thousands of the company's sales representatives to doctors, who then prescribed to the public.

Another approved substance was aspartame, but Mike Wallace in 1996 stated on his television program that the approval of aspartame was the most contested in FDA history. It is everywhere and in so many products we buy. In my opinion, it should be used sparingly or not at all.

After a drug is approved by the Federal Food and Drug Administration, a company cannot promote or sell it for any purposes other than those in its drug application. Doctors, however, can prescribe drugs for so-called off-label uses. Drug companies encourage doctors to prescribe drugs for new groups of patients. A change in this law would be very helpful to the public.

The promotion of drugs included in what Troy attorney Monica Navarro called "bogus studies" with as few as five patients to tout Topamax's other uses, and grants of as much as ten thousand dollars for doctors chosen as "thought leaders" to promote the drug for non-epilepsy uses. A grant is another meaning for offering free trips, dinners, or anything to get the doctors to prescribe the drug to their patients. Can you imagine what repercussions might happen to those poor children or adults who took this drug? It makes me sick just thinking about it. This is another example of a carefully calculated campaign of GREED.

In another example of promoting a drug for an unapproved use, Allergan Inc., the maker of wrinkle-smoothing Botox, just settled for six hundred million dollars for misbranding in their marketing. They led physicians to use Botox for uses like headache, pain, spasticity, and cerebral palsy in children? Children? Come on.

Don't get me wrong. The drug companies can be wonderful and have saved many lives, but they are not perfect, and as I have stated in a small amount of research provided here, in many cases their tests are flawed, many times in their favor. In some cases, ten years after the fact or thirty years later, people start dying or getting serious health problems from medications. Always read the side effects of the drugs you take. Most people just trust their doctors and take any drugs they prescribe. You should never take a drug unless you have done your own homework. With computers today, you or a friend can look up your drugs in a second and have every question answered. Check with your pharmacy to see if your prescription interacts with any other drugs you are taking. The doctors are so busy that they may not have time to check thoroughly.

It drives me crazy when you see an advertisement on television referring to some drug; legally, they must state the side effects, so they casually mention that you could get bowel problems, diarrhea, breathing problems, leaky urine, or die. Why would you take a drug with those side effects? Doctors all have their own ideas about treating disease. I prefer trying to heal with knowledge and changing lifestyles first. I could go on and on about drugs pulled off the market that are proven to be dangerous, but I think you get the picture.

I was diagnosed with very low vitamin D, which is the reason I went to a nutritionist. The body uses sunlight to manufacture vitamin D. I was shocked because I am a golfer plus I walk outdoors almost every day, so how could that be? I realized that they recently lowered their standards, as they did with cholesterol testing. My girlfriend, who has golfed for over thirty years, was also diagnosed with very low D. My wonderful daughter, who is getting so smart, told me not to get just any vitamin, but get a high-quality vitamin D. My doctor told me to take one thousand I.U. of D daily, and my girlfriend's doctor told her to take five hundred I.U. of vitamin D daily. Because of the difference in what the doctors said, I thought this was a perfect time to have a consultation with a nutritionist.

This nutritionist came very highly recommended to me. I had his name and number in my cell phone two years before I used it. I made the appointment and took my recent blood tests. His suggestion was that I take *five thousand* I.U., five days a week, and off on the weekends. My daughter is so smart (thanks, Nikki). After three months, I now have perfect vitamin D results.

The older I get the more of a naturalist I become.

*discipline is power*

chapter 22:

# GIVING BACK

*discipline is power*

∽

In her book, *The Angels and Me*, Elaine M. Grohman wrote "*Not by words alone do we reveal who we are.*"

My Father had AB negative blood, the rarest of blood types and donated regularly. I wanted to carry on his tradition and found out years ago, when I was pregnant, that I had O-negative blood. This blood type is carried by only 3 percent of the population and is universal. Having universal blood means my blood can be given to people with any blood type. I like having the kind of blood that can go to anyone. It's a special feeling.

I was a regular blood donor for years, and then all of a sudden, my iron count dropped, and they wouldn't take my blood anymore. I was very puzzled as to why this suddenly happened. I kept trying to give but was always rejected. So I started taking iron pills and went back a few months later to try to donate again. Still, I encountered rejection, rejection, and more rejection. I checked with my doctor to see if I could take more iron, and she said yes. I would keep trying to give blood, but still they would reject me. I checked with my doctor a second time to see if it was all right to take a triple dose of iron, and she said yes. A few months later, I tried to donate again and was rejected. I was starting to get a complex—I hate rejection!

Now, I was up to six iron pills a day; my stool was as black as night, and my iron levels were not increasing. So much for getting vitamins and minerals in pill form. One of the nurses who tested me said she wasn't supposed to tell me, but maybe if I ate more red meat, it would help. Her experiences showed that iron pills didn't do the job. She only told me this because I was whining that I was unable to donate for a very long time.

The first three months on the modified Atkins program, my hemoglobin jumped from thirty-six to forty-two, and they took my blood. I was happy again. I was on the low-fat, no-protein diet when they wouldn't take my blood, and what I learned from this lesson is that a week or two before I give blood, I eat red meat three or four times. I always try to eat naturally grass-fed, not corn-fed, antibiotic-injected beef.

Everyone should try to give blood a few times a year. It is just the right thing to do, and one of the nurses told me that it is healthy for you. Saving lives is good karma.

Find a way to give back. It makes you feel great. Do hospital work, work with kids, and give blood. Do anything for your fellow human beings. It is a selfish thing, too, because you feel so good doing it.

For the last fifteen years, I have volunteered at my local hospital, and I love it. I see old friends who come in for surgery, and I love the nurses and doctors with whom I work. What an amazing group of people. I know that I make a difference, and that is a tremendous feeling. *I make a difference.* Recently a friend and neighbor came in to my hospital for a double mastectomy at the young age of forty-five, and I was blessed that she was in my unit and I was able to give support to her and her family. She calls me her guardian angel. What a tragedy to undergo this type of health trauma at such a young age. Being able to give back is a tremendous feeling. I am happy to report she is doing well and almost finished with her treatment. God bless you girl!

The funny thing is people always ask me why I volunteer, and then they say, "Gee, I think I would like to volunteer, too." It gets people thinking about how to give back. They think I am special because I volunteer, but the real reason I do it is because I am selfish. I just feel good doing it and am very proud of my volunteer uniform and all my pins. The pins are for hours of service and my blood donations. Each time you donate, they give you a very creative pin for your lapel, and they look great on my uniform!

*discipline is power*

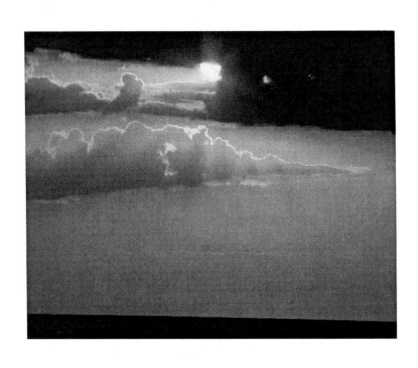

# chapter 23:

# FRIENDS AND LOVERS

*discipline is power*

∽

Friends are wonderful when they are wonderful people, and lovers can be amazing when they are amazing friends. Friends can even be like family in some instances, and possibly if you have children, when they move away and go off on their own, your friends will become as close as family.

Unfortunately, too many of us have hangers-on. The trouble with hangers-on is that they never go away until we are brave enough to send them away. They will kind of be there when you think you need them and all the while it's not real. They stay for sex, fame, jealousy, or maybe because they have no one else, but all the while they are not really there. It's not real. The bad part is that you can sense something is not right with this friend or lover and choose not to listen.

The issue here is if you choose to listen to your gut, it will tell you who **should** be a friend or lover. Your gut is what I refer to as the sixth sense (the first five senses are sight, hearing, touch, smell, and taste). If I had learned to listen to my gut when I was in my teens or twenties, I would have made far fewer mistakes.

In my experience, our dearest friends last for approximately a decade or so, then they move, we move, get divorced, or some kind of change takes place. I have reconnected with a very close friend from my early twenties in the last year or so, and childhood friends, and it was just as if we'd spoken every month or so—not some forty years later.

You know the old saying Keep your friends close but keep your enemies closer? That way you can watch them. My mom loved that saying. The decision of whether they stay or go is up to you. Be strong and make a decision. Know also that, as you age, you get smarter and more confident, which means that your decision making gets better and better. Learn to cultivate that sixth sense. Thankfully, something within your body moves up rather than drooping down.

If you are in a relationship that is going anywhere but where you want it to go, move along. I was told by an old friend (and I love this saying), "Men/women are like buses. Wait five minutes and another one comes along." Isn't that a great saying? We are looking for good husbands and good wives, not to own or be owned. This is why we have the dating process.

We sometimes stay in relationships because we are afraid of change. Look back at your life and, in hindsight, you can see where change has always promoted growth of some sort. You should learn something from every relationship Let your guts help guide you.

I left my first husband thirty-something times and always came back because I wanted it to work—no other reason. How stupid! It never worked from day one, but I wanted it to work, so I kept going back. I never wanted to disappoint my parents by getting divorced. Oh, horrors, a divorce! I have one brother who has been married four times, and the other will soon be married three times. One more divorce wouldn't have made any difference to my parents. Actually, my children are much better people because of my divorce and because of my present wonderful husband. I am also mother and friend to his three terrific adult children. The moral of this section is to pick your friends wisely and your lovers carefully… and if your sixth sense is talking to you, **LISTEN!**

*discipline is power*

# chapter 24:

# PHOTOSHOP PICTURES

*discipline is power*

∾

I think that I look fairly good at sixty-four, but want you to know that I work hard at trying to be the best I can be. I like being informed, so I read about things I am interested in. I work out hard and expend a tremendous amount of energy, so that I can have some fun eating and drinking, in moderation, of course. I am also somewhat of a camera buff, as you can see by all the pictures, but I learned something very interesting from my son-in-law, David. He has a new camera with a huge lens, and he is very good with computers. I feel he should be a professional photographer. He took the pictures for this book, and when we put them on his computer, he Photoshopped them.

*Photoshopped* is a term that I knew existed but I never *really* knew what it meant until I saw it firsthand. This is why all the covers of all the magazines with stars on them look so good. Every star looks unbelievable—because they *are* unbelievable! They are flawless, and they make us feel decrepit and ugly. Here is a secret that not everyone knows. They ARE all fake. The partially naked pictures, the close-ups, and the faraway body shots are all fake.

When David showed me how he was going to make me look so good, I couldn't believe it. I lost ten years on my face, and if I can have it done as a novice, the stars can do it with all their professional helpers. He didn't do anything to change my body structure, but if I wasn't happy with the body shot, he could have shaved my hips or thighs. I will never trust a magazine picture again. Even motion pictures can be edited in the postproduction phase.

This is just a reminder to show us that perfection is not realistic. Go to *google photoshop before and after* and you will see some of the pictures I am referring to.

I am concerned that all of our teenagers and young adults are comparing themselves to these fake photographs. I am told that all the top fashion magazines are using Photoshop. Finally, they are exposed! Tell your children and show them the before-and-after pictures.

*discipline is power*

# in closing

❧

I recently read a paragraph Jim Beglen, an acquaintance of mine, wrote:

> What I've learned is that, although life is a one-way ticket, the aging route is not a straight line. There are twists, turns, speed bumps, hills, and sometimes mountains along the way. How we travel the route, and how we react to challenges, has a great deal to do with the quality of the trip.

**I thought he put it perfectly.**

I wanted to put some of my experiences into a tool for learning, for anyone who is interested. Experience is a great teacher, and it is important for me to pass along information that might be helpful or enhance someone's life.

One of the most important people in my life, my younger brother, the heavier smoker, has had a series of ministrokes and, thankfully, is recovering as I write this. He is very special to me, and now I know he will listen to my words of warning. He will learn how to change his life and get to the incredible, healthy future he desires and desperately wants. You can, too. Remember, **you find out what you are made of in the face of adversity**.

Fast-forward a year, and he is a non smoker for almost a year. I am so proud of him.

Oh, the other brother met a girl who really doesn't care for him smoking his ten crummy cigarettes a week. I am so grateful to her because he quit, too (thanks, Fe!). So both brothers have quit, along with my newest sister-in-law, Tina. Oh, joy!

Right now, right this minute, write down your **wants and needs**. Put them into affirmations and get going on a whole new positive, smarter, and more confident you, who knows exactly what you **want and need**. And, remember, **to be good at anything, love, eat, sleep, and breathe it.** Please start today...

I won't say good luck because I know that if you believe, you will have good luck. Then your wants and needs will come to you.☺

WANTS AND NEEDS:

———————————————————————
———————————————————————
———————————————————————
———————————————————————
———————————————————————
———————————————————————
———————————————————————
———————————————————————
———————————————————————

BELIEVE IN YOURSELF!
Some of my very favorite quotes are:
"The universe has an uncanny ability to weave the events long before they arrive."—Elaine Grohman.

"The only thing that stands between a person and what they want from life is often the will to try and the faith to believe it's possible."—Rick DeVoss

"You are today where your thoughts brought you; you will be tomorrow where your thoughts take you."—James Allen

"Luck is a by product of hard work."—Todd Matthews

"Giving love and getting love makes a happier person."—Lola Sinelli

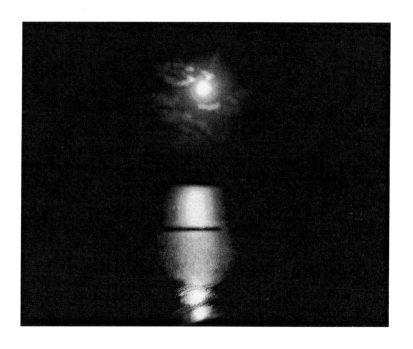

# bibliography

❧

Chapter 1: *ColorMe Beautiful  Carole Jackson 1980 Acropolis Books ltd, 1980*
Chapter 4: Dr. Stanley Gulin, MD Board Certified Plastic Surgeon, Naples Florida

Chapter 5: *1.About.com: Dermatology*
Chapter 5: published in the April 2010 issue of *Archives of Dermatology*, a journal of the American Medical Association.
Chapter 5: Puritans pride ads by google

Chapter 7: Wikipedia, calorie Professor Haub, CNN Health.com November 8, 2010

Chapter 8: Harvard Health Publications 9/10/2010
Chapter 8: Time to run.com 9/10/2010

Chapter 8: William Dufty, Sugar Blues, 1975 Clinton Book Co.
Chapter 8: Ann Louise Gittleman, How to Stay Young and Healthy in a Toxic World copywright Keats Publishing 1999

Chapter 9: BPA New York Times dated April 16, 2008

Chapter 13: The Fantastic Voyage by Ray Kurzweil and
Terry Grossman M.D. 2004 Holtz Brinch Publishers
Chapter 14: The Detroit Free Press Sept 2, 2010

Chapter 15: Dr. Isadore Rosenfeld Doctor, what should
I eat. Copywright 1995 Isadore Rosenfeld
Chapter 15: about.com, alcohol beverages on low carb
diet National institutes of health webside dated 9.4.10
       Dr. Isadore Rosenfeld Doctor, what should I
       eat copywright 1995 Isadore Rosenfeld
       National Institutes of Health website dated
       9/4/2010

Chapter 16: Center for Disease Control
       Health Magazine May 2009
       Ezine Articles by Google 9/10/20
       Dr. Mercola January 26, 2010 email
       Lab test online, June 18, 2010

Chapter 17: Wikipedia, the free encyclopedia
       Dr. William Gutierreez, D.C.
       About.com Thyroid Disease
       Dr. Oz, Womans World June 2010
       Dr. William Gutierreez, D.C.
       Ask.com

Chapter 18: Dr. Atkins New Diet Revolution, copywright
1992 Harper Collins

Chapter 20:  About.com
       About.com

Chapter 21: HealingWell.com, Dr. William Cockburn
Dr. William Gutierreez, D.C., Nutriotionist, Doctor of Chiropractic Medicine
Dr. J. Stuart Wolf, University of Michigan Hospital
Janette 'D. Sherman, Md, Life's Delicate Balance, copywright 2000 Publisher Taylor and Francis
Dr. David E. Goldberg, PhD, chief of Genetic Epidemiology Group at the International Agency for Research on Cancer , Lyon, France.
*Experience Magazine*, May 2010,


Chapter 22: Det *What Your Doctor May Not Tell You About Menopause*, by Dr. John R. Lee with Virginia Hopkins, 1996 Cr, Warner Books
Dr. Mercola, Reliable Answers News and Commentary by Debbi Pearl
Dana Ullman, who is an author of ten books on homeopathic medicine, owner, Homiopathic Educational Services
*The Truth about Drug Companies: How They Deceive Us and What to Do About It*, Dr. Marcia Angell, who was the former editor-in-chief of the *New England Journal of Medicine*,
2005, Dr. John Ioannidis, an epidemiologist at Ioannina School of Medicine, Greece, , why most published research findings are false, 2008, Dr. Ioannidis again showed that much of "scientific research being published is highly questionable

*May 25, 2010, in the Detroit Free Press*
*Mike Wallace, Febuary 9, 2010 Coca Cola a closer look Mike Wallace June 17th 2008 Brain Cancer and FDA approval*
*Monica Navarro Bogus studies, May 25, 2010 Detroit Free Press*
*Allergan, Pharma September 8, 2010, September blog*

*Chapter 23:* Elaine M. Grohman's book, *The Angels and Me*